Physical Therapy Administration and Management

Second Edition

Physical Therapy Administration and Management

Second Edition

ROBERT J. HICKOK

Coordinating Editor

Assistant Vice Chancellor of Medical Affairs
Washington University School of Medicine
St. Louis, Missouri

Published for The American Physical
Therapy Association by

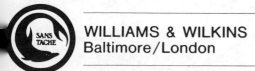

WILLIAMS & WILKINS
Baltimore/London

Copyright © 1982
Williams & Wilkins
428 E. Preston Street
Baltimore, Md. 21202, U.S.A.

Made in the United States of America
First Edition, July 1974
Reprinted August 1975
Reprinted October 1978
Reprinted August 1979
Reprinted February 1981

Library of Congress Cataloging in Publication Data

Physical therapy administration and management.

    Includes index.
    Contents: Personnel management/Jack M. Hofkosh—Policies and procedures/ James Rood-house—Departmental planning, design and construction/Charles M. Magistro—[etc.]
    1. Physical therapy services—Administration. I. Hickok, Robert J., 1926–   . II. American Physical Therapy Association (1921–)
RM713.P58 1982   362.1'78   82-2003
ISBN 0-683-03976-8   AACR2

Composed and printed at the
Waverly Press, Inc.
Mt. Royal and Guilford Aves.
Baltimore, Md. 21202, U.S.A.

FOREWORD

The first edition of *Physical Therapy Administration and Management* was a milestone publication. It represented an initial effort to produce a comprehensive text and reference directed specifically to the administrative and management facets of a physical therapy service. The need for this book was made self-evident by the number of volumes sold. Its existence is a credit to those many volunteers who served as authors and reviewers, giving unselfishly of themselves and working in an atmosphere of some critics who were saying "It can't be done!"

This new second edition has enriched significantly the first effort and speaks well to the growth and sophistication of the management aspects of physical therapy. High praise is deserved by all who have contributed to this project.

Royce P. Noland
Executive Director
American Physical Therapy Association

PREFACE to the First Edition

A need exists in physical therapy literature for a comprehensive review of administrative and management techniques that relate specifically to physical therapists. It is the intent of this book to fill this need.

An almost universal indictment of the health care industry has been its timidity in adopting contemporary administrative practices. Physical therapy has followed, to some extent, the models set by other health professions and health care institutions, i.e., a rightful and long-standing concern for educational and patient care standards. To indicate, however, that physical therapists have not addressed themselves to the administrative problems inherent in an increasingly complex health care system is in error. In the period from 1965 to 1970, almost 80 articles exploring all facets of administration have appeared in the Journal of the American Physical Therapy Association

The advent of medicare, medicaid, and the prospect of national health insurance has served to focus further attention on the need to hone administrative skills. Long the custodian of a small subdivision of a general hospital, the physical therapist has moved to a variety of treatment settings such as home health services, skilled nursing facilities, rehabilitation centers, private practice, and public health programs. The expansion of treatment settings has not ended. Now emerging are prepaid group practices such as Health Maintenance Organizations which pose new challenges to the physical therapist. In these multiple settings, the physical therapist must be able to provide not only excellence in patient care but also equal skill in understanding and implementing the business aspects of a service.

This book builds on the earlier work, expands and deepens the quality of information, and provides one central source of information on administrative aspects of physical therapy. Since administrative and management problems are quite similar in all organizations regardless of the end product, this book does not delve deeply into the theoretical and philosophical aspects of administration, since a vast body of knowledge has been amassed on this subject. The presentation is a pragmatic, problem-solving approach relating specifically to the problems unique to physical therapists. It is directed toward clinicians, students, health care administrators, physicians, educators, and department managers. In short, it is designed as a resource for health care workers who need more knowledge about physical therapy administrative practices.

The content of the book has been divided into seven interest areas which cover various aspects of administration, including medico-legal problems and departmental design.

This book brings into focus and creates interest in matters frequently considered dull or, at best, bureaucratic chores. We believe that excellence in patient care, the essential purpose for our existence, can be achieved when carried out with sensitivity to and appreciation of sound administrative and management principles.

Robert J. Hickok

ACKNOWLEDGMENTS

I would like to express my sincere appreciation to Eugene Michels, Associate Executive Director of the American Physical Therapy Association for his assistance to the editor and the contributing authors in the production of this second edition. Mr. Michels, well accepted as the resident guru of writing for Physical Therapists, gave freely of his time and considerable talent to significantly focus and sharpen the language of this second edition. I know the contributing authors join me in thanking Eugene Michels for his assistance.

Robert J. Hickok

CONTRIBUTORS

Armour, James A, Director of Quality Assurance, The Mercy Hospital of Pittsburgh, Pittsburgh, Pennsylvania

Hofkosh, Jack M., Director, Physical Therapy, Institute of Rehabilitation Medicine, New York, New York

Horsh, Donald J., Associate Director, Graduate Program in Health Care Administration, Washington University School of Medicine, St. Louis, Missouri

Magistro, Charles M., Director of Physical Therapy, Pomona Valley Community Hospital, Pomona, California

McKillip, James B., Director, Valley Physical Therapy Center, Van Nuys, California

Roodhouse, James W., Administrator, Institute of Physical Medicine and Rehabilitation, Peoria, Illinois

Savander, Gary R., Vice President, Hamilton Physical Therapy Services, P.A., Trenton, New Jersey

Wessman, Henry C., Associate Professor and Chairman, Department of Physical Therapy, University of North Dakota School of Medicine, Grand Forks, North Dakota

CONTENTS

INTRODUCTION

In the early 1970s, the American Physical Therapy Association was faced with the dilemma of having to decide whether to participate in the re-issuance of a brief monograph on Physical Therapy Administration or to undertake the publication of a more comprehensive document to better serve the needs of Physical Therapists. The latter course was chosen and in 1974, the book *Physical Therapy Administration and Management* was published.

In the preface to the first edition, it was stated that "a need exists in physical therapy literature for a comprehensive review of administrative and management techniques that relate specifically to physical therapists. It is the intent of this book to fill this void."

In retrospect it was naive to consider the first edition or the current second edition as a comprehensive review of administrative and management techniques. More realistically, the book *Physical Therapy Administration and Management* has served as a major source of basic information regarding Physical Therapy Administration and Management. Its success has been attested to by the sustained sale of the book for the past 8 years.

To provide a setting for the chapters to follow, it seems important to examine the "climate" or "environment" that exists in the Health Care Industry—to look first at the conditions that modified the administrative environment; then to examine the response of the field of Physical Therapy to these changes. Webster defines environment as "that which environs, surroundings, specifically the aggregate of all external conditions and influences affecting life and the development of an organism, human behavior, society and etc (1)." If we focus on the "aggregate of all external conditions," then an approach is available to analyze the administrative environment of the past, look at the present, and to be predictive of the future. Certainly, the external conditions of the past 20 years presented more turbulence, more sociological unrest, more technological advance, and more sweeping change in the way health care was financed, delivered, and administered than in any comparable period in history.

The evolution of the administrative environment that exists in health care today can be brought into focus by looking at the hospital as an organizational model. During the early years of the 20th century hospitals were simple organizations, often characterized as examples of a "cottage industry." The business aspects of a hospital were often handled by Boards of Trustees who divided the duties—finance, physical plant and so forth. A nurse was often designated as superintendent. Physicians did not need the hospital since he saw his private patients in his office. Hospitals were feared by a majority of people and often became a repository of the indigent.

During the 1920s, medicine began to dominate. The explosion that took place in scientific medicine changed the needs of the physician, making him dependent on the hospital. The mystique of medicine, combined with charisma of the physician, gave him a dominating role in an increasingly larger, more complex institution.

The emergence of Administration as a force in the hospital was of more recent vintage. It gained momentum following World War II. The period from 1946 to the early 1960s was a relatively untroubled time during which the experiences of the second World War were being translated to civilian use. As an example, there was the emergence of Rehabilitation as a health care movement in which restorative care was organized into comprehensive programs with Medicine, Physical Therapy, Occupational Therapy, Nursing, Social Work, and others working in a "team" concept of care. This movement provided the opportunity for physical therapists to begin migrating from the hospital setting. During this period, as well, the Hill-Burton Hospital Construction Act of 1946 provided federal dollars for the construction of many new hospitals, frequently in rural America. Again, new opportunities were created for physical therapists to practice. There was a slow but steady integration of new technology into the health care work place, both in clinical practice and in the application of more sophisticated administrative practices. And, the third party payer, i.e., Blue Cross, Blue Shield, and others became universally accepted as the way to finance institutional health care needs. The increasing complexity of the hospital; the proliferation of new health professions; the impact of the Joint Commission on Accreditation of Hospitals, all tended to propel "Administration" into a more prominent role on the hospital scene. "Administration" received a major thrust into prominence with the entry of the Federal Government into health care in a massive way with the enactment of Medicare legislation on July 1, 1965 (2).

THE IMPACT OF FEDERAL PROGRAMS

The impact of Medicare was pervasive triggering service demands on a health system already functioning at near capacity. With the passage of Medicare legislation, the federal government instituted a major marketing effort to enhance public acceptance and use of the new programs. As an example, within two years after Medicare was implemented, over 2,000 Home Health Agencies were organized and operating. Extended Care Facilities (now Skilled Nursing Facilities) were rushed to completion, with an anticipated deluge of patients over the age of 65. Hospitals also responded to this federal prodding, and with 30 to 40 percent of their income assured, began extensive building programs; upgraded salaries and accelerated the use of contemporary administrative/management practices to deal with complex governmental regulations that accompanied Medicare.

The response of the health care industry during the period federal programs were initiated can be illustrated by looking at national health expenditures since 1940 (3) (see Table I.1). In 1940, the gross national product was $100 billion, of which $4 billion was spent on Health, or 4 percent of the total GNP. And, during the period from 1940 to 1960, the percent of GNP spent on health went from 4 percent to 5.3 percent, a modest increase. From 1960 to 1980, the percent of the GNP spent on health jumped an additional 4.1 percent to 9.4 percent. Whether this significant increase in the commitment of our national resources to health care can be attributed to medicare is debatable. What cannot be debated is that Medicare, by the magnitude of the program, served as the keystone of federal initiatives that contributed heavily to the circumstance that close to 10 percent of the GNP is being committed to health care services.

Accompanying Medicare were other key pieces of legislation that contributed to the administrative environment of today. The Partnership in Health Act (Public Law 89–749) was passed in 1966 and provided for the development of state and area wide comprehensive health planning agencies (4). The intent was to bring order out of chaos; to attack the nonsystem of the health care industry by "voluntary" planning; to restructure the system to eliminate duplication and fragmentation of services, and to coordinate the flow of health services in a coherent manner. Also deeply imbedded in the fabric of this legislation was the concept of "consumerism," i.e., the right of the consumer to have a major role in planning for health services. The concept of consumerism epitomized the social turmoil and sociological change that accompanied the great society legislation of the 1960s. However, the attempt at voluntary planning was largely a failure, and Comprehensive Health Planning Agencies, without effective power, were frequently ignored.

During this same period an ambitious program was devised to translate the results of research in heart disease, cancer, and stroke came into existence

Table I.1
National Health Expenditures 1940–1980

Year	Gross National Product (GNP)	Health Care Costs	Percent of GNP
	billion	*billion*	
1940	100	4	4.0
1950	286.5	12.7	4.4
1960	506.5	26.9	5.3
1970	997.7	74.7	7.5
1980	2,627.1	247.2	9.4

(5). Known as Regional Medical Programs, this effort flowered briefly, was deemed a failure by congress, and put out of existence.

As governmental health programs gained momentum, spiraling costs became the deep concern of federal legislators. Where the 1960s was a period of expansion, the 1970s became the period of "regulation." Programs that were force fed into existence were faced with a formidable weapon, "retroactive denial of payment." Continued concern about costs and quality of care produced additional legislation that has had and is continuing to have a profound effect on the way health professions deliver care. Comprehensive Health Planning Agencies have been replaced by Health Systems Agencies; the illusion of voluntary planning disappeared. Health Systems Agencies have to approve any capital expenditure over $600,000 and in most areas Certificates of Need have to be obtained before construction of health facilities can proceed.

One of the most provocative legislative actions taken in the last decade was Public Law 92-603 (6), which amended the Medicare provisions of the Social Security Act. Two sections are worthy of comment. Section 251-c introduced the principle of salary equivalency. A concept that tied reimbursement to the median salary of an employed health professional in a given region, as determined by the Department of Labor. Section 251-c is of concern to physical therapists because they were specifically identified as a professional group. Its real significance was that it proposed a new approach to reimbursement that challenged the "fee for service" principle, which was dominant in the provision of a broad range of health care services.

Section 249-c set forth provisions for the development of Professional Standards Review Organizations. This section (PSRO) was based on the premise that health professionals are the most appropriate individuals to evaluate the quality of medical services and that Peer Review at the local level is the soundest method of assuring the appropriate use of health resources and facilities.

The Professional Standards Review section called for PSROs to review the health care provided under Medicare, Medicaid, Maternal Child Health Programs, and Crippled Children's Programs and to make judgments on the medical necessity and the quality of care. In addition, PSROs were to determine whether care was being provided at a level which is most economical and consistent with the patient's medical care needs. Both sections represented the apex of the regulatory thrust of the federal government of the 1970s as a strategy to contain costs while publicizing the quality assurance aspect of the program.

The reaction to the PSROs has been extensive, and all professional health organizations with members involved in direct patient care have responded with new approaches to Quality Assurance assessment. Physical therapists have responded, as well, and Chapter 7 will provide a detailed treatment of the subject.

However, with the 1980s, a mood of conservatism prevailed throughout the country. The continuing upward spiral of health care costs, which were accelerating at a rate about one and one-half times greater than other segments of the economy, brought about a series of proposals in congress to deregulate the health care industry, the perception being that competition would close marginal institutions and the remaining facilities would compete in the free market place for patients. Congress hoped for a result, a lowering of health care costs, or at a minimum, a reduction in the rate of cost escalation. By January 1982 the instruments of "regulation" were being dismantled. Health Systems Agencies were being phased out, and Professional Standards Review Organizations were under serious attack. The era of "deregulation" was upon us. At this printing it is not clear how deregulation of the health care industry will end, but, clearly, the environment in which we practice will be substantially changed.

RESPONSE OF PHYSICAL THERAPY

During this period of governmental incursion, technological change, and a rapidly rising expectation by the public for health services, the field of Physical Therapy underwent a striking transformation. The magnitude of this transformation with its pronounced effect on clinical and administrative practices can be illustrated by looking at some key indicators in the time frame from 1950 to 1980: number of educational programs, work settings; number of practitioners; and the size of communities in which physical therapists practice.

EDUCATIONAL PROGRAMS

A review of the journal *Physical Therapy* revealed that in 1950 there were 28 accredited schools offering programs in physical therapy training. These were primarily bachelors of science and certificate programs. The number increased to 38 in 1960; by 1970, 51 undergraduate and certificate programs were in existence, with an additional 11 offering a graduate degree. By 1980, the number of undergraduate programs reached 78, with 21 graduate degree programs in operation. Of interest, and of real significance, was the fact that 54 programs were training physical therapists assistants, a category of workers that did not exist until the late 1960s. By 1980, in the aggregate, there were 153 programs offering training programs ranging from the associate degree for the Physical Therapist's Assistant to the Doctorate in Physical Therapy.

WORK SETTINGS

At the close of World War II, it was a generally accepted "rule of thumb" that close to 85 percent of all physical therapists worked in acute hospitals. This serves to dramatize the recent findings of a membership profile survey by the American Physical Therapy Association (7). The study results recorded 14 separate facilities in which physical therapists worked. Also recorded was a cumulative "other" category which included 3 percent of the sample (see Table I.2). It is of interest to highlight some of these data. Less than 50 percent of physical therapists now work in acute hospitals. And, 10 percent are in private practice. Other significant work sites are Rehabilitation Centers, 9 percent; Extended Care Facility/Nursing Home, 8 percent; Home Health Agencies, 6 percent; Public or nonpublic schools, 6 percent, and Academic Institutions provided employment for 5 percent of the respondents. A variety of other settings provided a work setting for 2 percent or less. This supports the contention that physical therapists have greatly diversified their employment sites in response to changing societal needs.

NUMBER OF PRACTITIONERS

Active membership in the American Physical Therapy Association appears to be a reasonable measure of growth that can be generalized to all physical therapists. In 1950, there were 3374 physical therapists with active membership in the American Physical Therapy Association (8). By 1960 the number had grown to 6242, an 85 percent increase. And, by 1970 an additional 75

Table I.2
Type of Facility or Institution in Which Salaried and Self-Employed Do Most or All of Work ($N = 12,344$)[a]

Facility	N	Percent
Hospital	5801	47
Private office	1222	10
Rehabilitation center	1138	9
Extended care facility/ nursing home	1010	8
Home health agency	724	6
Public or non-public school	696	6
Academic institution	640	5
Specialty clinic	206	2
Residential care facility	188	2
Governmental department or agency	178	2
Voluntary health agency	51	0
Prepaid health care organization	48	0
Research centers	23	0
Industry	13	0
Other	377	3
Total	12,315	100

(No response 29)

[a] Source; The American Physical Therapy Association, Membership Profile Survey, January 1979.

percent increase occurred and the total reached 10,919. A precipitous increase of 142 percent occurred in the decade ending in 1980 with 26,428 members in the active membership category.

SIZE OF COMMUNITIES

As to the size communities in which physical therapists practice, there is a rather even distribution throughout the country (see Table I.3). Twenty-nine percent of physical therapists practice in communities of less than 50,000 population and 19 percent in communities of one million or more, with a rather even spread in the four other size communities listed (7) (see Table I.3). The surprise here is the concentration of physical therapists in communities of less than 50,000. This runs counter to a normally accepted perception that health professionals, in general, gravitate to our larger population centers, but confirms that physical therapists have moved aggressively to meet service needs wherever they may be.

In summary, the field of Physical Therapy emerged from this 30-year period as a major health profession with a five-fold increase in accredited educational programs; a seven-fold increase in active membership in the American Physical Therapy Association; dispersion to 14 significant work sites and migration rather evenly to communities of all sizes; and, above all, with many new requirements for expertise in administration and management as well as an expanding clinical role in providing health services.

CONCLUSION

This second edition of the book *Physical Therapy Administration and Management* has undergone substantial changes to meet contemporary needs. One chapter was dropped, and a new chapter (Five) on quality assurance added. The new chapter briefly traces the history of quality assurance as a concept,

Table I.3
Population Size of Cities in Which Salaried and Self-Employed Do Most or All of Work (N = 12,344)[a]

Population	n	Percent
1,000,000 or more	2,371	19
500,000–999,999	1,522	12
250,000–499,999	1,183	10
100,000–249,999	1,662	14
50,000–99,999	1,902	16
Under 50,000	3,559	29
Total	12,199	100
(No response 145)		

[a] Source, The American Physical Therapy Association, Membership Profile Survey, January 1979.

and presents a method for accruing statistics using a computer based software program as a basis for monitoring care. A program for assessing the results of care is presented which includes the development of screening criteria. This chapter substantially addresses the major concern brought about by the climate of regulation of the 1970s. Chapter five's content should provide a framework for dealing with the changing requirements of the Joint Commission on Accreditation of Hospitals and other regulatory bodies.

The remaining chapters—Records, Personnel Management, Fiscal Management, Policies and Procedures, Departmental Planning, and Design—have been rigorously updated and in some cases substantially changed to reflect the administration/management climate of today. And, as indicated previously, the thrust of the book remains the same—a source of general information on Administration/Management to meet the needs of clinicians, students, health care administrators, physicians, educators, and department managers.

Robert J. Hickok

References

1. *Webster's New Collegiate Dictionary*, Eighth Edition. A. Merriam-Webster, G & C Merriam Co., Sringfield, Mass. 382
2. Social Security Act of 1965 (PL 89–97).
3. Gibson, Robert M., and Waldo, Daniel R.: National Health Expenditure, 1980, Health Financing Review, Vol. 3, No. 1, Sept 1981, pp. 1–54.
4. The Comprehensive Health Planning and Public Health Service Amendment Acts of 1966 (PL 89–749).
5. The Heart, Cancer and Stroke Amendments of 1965 (PL 89–239).
6. Terenzio, J. V.: The National Health Planning and Resources Act of 1974, Bulletin of the New York Academy of Medicine 52 (December 1976) 1236.
7. The American Physical Therapy Association *Membership Profile Survey*, January 1979.
8. Garrett, Gary R. Associate Director, Department of Professional Services, American Physical Therapy Association: Personal communication.

chapter 1

PERSONNEL MANAGEMENT

Jack M. Hofkosh

Managers, supervisors, and personnel are people. People make up and carry out the work of organizations. Hospitals and other health care agencies are organizations. Personnel management in physical therapy is management of people, by people, in organizations.

These few opening sentences set the perspective, purpose, and scope of this chapter. The emphasis is on the human behavior aspects of organizations, management, and work. Theory is balanced with observations based on my own experiences as a manager and supervisor and with practical suggestions for putting ideas to use.

An understanding of organizations is essential. In the health care industry, as in other industries, organizations have become larger, more complex, and more impersonal for the people who work within them. As size and complexity increase, individualism decreases, the scope of individual action narrows, central management becomes more isolated from middle management and other employees, and employees experience a growing alienation from their work and from the organization.

The content of this chapter is intended to help the physical therapist manager or supervisor understand and carry out his duties as a manager of people in organizational settings of any size or kind. The content should also be of interest and use in the prospective manager or supervisor and to anyone who works or will work in physical therapy: the staff physical therapist, the physical therapist assistant, the student, the secretary or clerk, and the physical therapy aide. Each is a person whose work and ideas are essential to the organization, and together they can influence the duties and style of the manager or supervisor.

ORGANIZATION

Any organization represents participation by a number of people in pursuit of a common goal, purpose, or mission (4). The mission is generally one that an individual could not accomplish alone and that requires the coordinated effort of the people who make up the organization (23, 24). Because of the required coordination, an organization usually has a division of labor or

1

departmentalization and a hierarchy of authority (23, 24, 31). The classical organization, when depicted in an organization chart or table of organization, is pyramidal, with centralized top management at the tip and work or service units at the base of the pyramid. An organization chart for a typical hospital can be found in Zimmerman's article (32).

The classical pyramidal structure of the typical organization continues to exist for two good reasons: clarity and stability (23). A great deal of attention has been given to how to make work in this structure more productive and more satisfying to employees, but nobody has devised an effective alternative to the basic pyramid.

Line Relationships

Line relationships, often referred to as the chain of command, are the vertical lines of authority and responsibility connecting each position with those above and below it in the organization. The specifics of line relationships in any organization, that is, which position is the superior and which the subordinate, are usually shown in the organization chart and stated in the organization's job descriptions. The physical therapist director, for example, may have direct line responsibility to a hospital administrator or to a director of clinical services, and, at the same time, may have direct line authority over supervisors of special units in the physical therapy department. In turn, these supervisors may have line authority over the staff—physical therapists, physical therapist assistants, and physical therapy aides—who work in the units.

The line relationships within a physical therapy department will, of course, vary with the size, complexity, and subdivisions (if any) of the department.

The vertical line relationships of authority and responsibility provide channels of upward and downward communication which are necessary but usually not enough to meet all of the communication needs of an organization. An organization chart that attempts to show not only the line relationships but all lines of communication for coordination, medical relations, administrative services, and records management, for example, could be so complex as to defy interpretation.

The line relationships, like the pyramidal structure, evolved as a way of not only organizing the efforts of people but also managing the people in the organization. Later sections of this chapter show, however, that managing people requires more than a division of labor and a hierarchy of authority. Some experts even say that the management problem is how to get the pyramidal structure to work in spite of itself (23).

ORGANIZATION GOALS

Every organization has, or should have, a statement of goals or objectives by which its performance can be measured. Whether broad and sweeping, as in a mission statement, or quite detailed, as in specific objectives, these goals are results-oriented and represent the reason for existence of the organization. Each unit, department, or program in the organization should have goals or objectives that are consistent with and contributory to those of the organization.

The content of the organization's goals will, of course, vary with the nature of the organization, the kinds of people who make it up, and the kinds of consumers who receive, use, or benefit from its services or products. Whether the content of the goals, a primary concern of management is productivity, that is, achievement of the goals in the most effective and efficient manner given the human, financial, and other resources available to the organization. Among the experts on organizations and among managers, there is no disagreement on productivity being a primary concern. The disagreement, where it exists, is over the methods used to increase productivity.

New technology and design of work space can increase productivity up to a point. Inherent in any organization is the fact that people carry out, supervise, and manage the work necessary for achieving the organization's goals. As in any labor-intensive organization, the problem in the hospital or the physical therapy department is how to manage people so as to obtain their commitment to the organization's goals and thereby increase productivity. The mounting evidence in industrial and organizational psychology indicates that employees who feel frustrated, threatened, and alienated at work form into informal groups whose goals run counter to the goals of management and organization (24).

Since about the middle of this century, participation in decision-making, job satisfaction, and personal growth in the job have become increasingly important in personnel management to increase productivity in achieving organization goals (1, 3, 23, 24). In the view of some individuals, these personnel factors are so important as to warrant being considered goals of the organization.

MANAGEMENT AND SUPERVISION

Managers are said to be those persons in an organization who have the power to make decisions (24). If one agrees with that simplified definition, then supervisors are those persons who oversee the work of others and presumably have no power to make decisions. Perhaps this distinction between managers and supervisors can be made in some large industrial or commercial organization, or even in some large health care settings, especially if one looks at the organization chart rather than at what managers and supervisors actually do.

The physical therapist who is director of a department usually has the power to make some decisions (e.g., hiring a particular person to fill a staff vacancy) but not others (e.g., raising the salary ranges for positions in the department). At the same time, this director may be responsible for overseeing the work of some or all of the personnel in the department. Zimmerman makes the point that supervision of personnel is basically a human relations skill, to be distinguished from the knowledges and skills required for management in terms of planning, organizing, budgeting, designing systems and procedures, scheduling, establishing job descriptions and work standards, and evaluating the service (29). Hickok includes most of the latter functions in the supervisor's role (11). Rather than trying to draw a hard line between management functions and supervision functions, this chapter recognizes that both kinds of functions may be the responsibility of the physical therapist director of a department. Also, the degree of management assumed by the physical therapist director may vary with that person's employment status, that is, as either a salaried employee or a contractor.

The terms of manager, supervisor, management, and supervision are used interchangeably in what follows, the intention being that everything discussed can be applicable to the physical therapist director of a department.

Supervisory Relationships and Roles

The supervisor may be called by various names, but the job in any enterprise is getting out production, maintaining quality performance, and serving as management's hand servant. The position has changed in the last 50 or so years as a result of adjustments in our social, political, and economic lives. Some of these adjustments occurred because of:

1. increasing size and complexity of the work place,
2. subdivisions of production,
3. unionization of subordinates,
4. technological and specialization functions,
5. social legislation, and
6. government incursions in the work place.

Some of the factors identified above have diminished the authority of the supervisor and enhnaced the positions of subordinates, and some have changed or made more complex the responsibilities of the supervisor.

The supervisor is caught between having to *report to* superiors in management and being a *representative of* management in relations to subordinates. This is no mean dilemma! The fact is that the supervisor is legally a part of management, receiving orders and directions from, and thus interacting in an upward manner with, members of management. He also interacts downward with subordinates. Another problem in this regard is the probability of his having been promoted from among the now subordinate group.

Because of these dilemmas there are at least five relationships that require the supervisor to play different roles:

1. living with oneself as an individual, that is, an *intra-personal* relationship;
2. forming a relationship with other supervisors as a peer group;

3. developing an authority-responsibility relationship with subordinates;
4. developing a relationship as a subordinate to superiors; and
5. being part of and dependent upon the wider culture in which one operates.

The intrapersonal relationship is a complex one in which emotions, beliefs, and many assumptions constitute what we are as human beings. The trained supervisor, to be truly successful, must believe in the concept that the intrinsic worth of the individual be understood and respected. As with all people, the supervisor experiences occasional incompatibility between reason and emotions. This intrapersonal relationship presents one of the larger problems that must be overcome if one is to function effectively as a supervisor.

The peer group relationship is based largely on friendship, assistance, encouragement, and acceptance. The supervisor depends on this acceptance sometimes even more than on approval from superiors.

The supervisor-subordinate relationships, perhaps the most important organizational relationships, are vertical and predicated upon the master-servant doctrine of common law. They include the concept that the supervisor has authority over subordinates and is responsible to a superior for their action. A supervisor's effectiveness depends upon using authority with discretion so as not to alienate subordinates. The subordinates must display discipline and be accountable for their actions as they assume responsibility by accepting a position in the organization. The supervisor, too, is under the control of a superior and has the duty of carrying out his or her responsibility to the superior in a loyal, enthusiastic, and sincere way.

The supervisor has a relationship as well with the wider culture in which he operates. The department and the hospital do not exist in a vacuum but in the total environment in which they are located. This total environment, known as the "social environment," is impacted from all sides by the many forces that are cause for change throughout our world of work.

The relationships and roles of the supervisor can be markedly influenced by collective bargaining and other labor relations activities, especially if these activities involve the physical therapist members of the staff (26). Just what the influence is depends upon the supervisor's decision to align himself or herself with the bargaining group or with administration or to refrain from taking any part in the negotiations (26). The supervisor who participates in these negotiations becomes adept at balancing the rights of subordinates, administrators, and the publics to be served and learns to recognize the need for the various regulations and adjustments and how to adapt to them.

The supervisor's relationships and roles will also be influenced by the educational and functional levels of the subordinates to be supervised. Supervising physical therapist assistants will be quite different from supervising physical therapy aides (13), and both of these situations will differ from supervising physical therapists (some of whom may themselves be supervisors) and secretarial or clerical staff.

Managerial and Supervisory Functions

Managers and supervisors have responsibility for certain functions that bear directly on personnel management and are considered in detail in later sections of this chapter: motivation, communications, recruitment and selection, performance appraisal, and retention and development. Other functions are presented briefly below, with descriptions taken chiefly from Hickok (11) and Zimmerman (29).

Planning includes establishing objectives and priorities, developing policies, determining methods and procedures, and scheduling implementation, all with an eye to charting the future course of the department.

Organizing is subdividing the total work to be done into jobs, duties, groups, and relationships, and delegating authority and responsibility.

Directing includes guiding, instructing, and persuading subordinates; establishing work standards; and making work assignments.

Cost analysis and budgeting, considered together here, include the retrospective review and prospective projection of objectives, activities, resources, expenditures, and income.

Evaluation, exclusive of performance appraisal, which is considered later, is the systematic study of the degree to which objectives are achieved and the reconsideration of objectives, priorities, policies, methods, and organizational structure. The results of this evaluation feed directly into planning.

Management must continuously be aware of new trends and technologies that will have impact on the effectiveness of managerial and supervisory functions. It must maintain a steady flow of tried and true methods, while at the same time allowing for innovations and creativity in the development of new ideas and methods and in the adoption of new technologies. Extreme fluctuations in methods, procedures, activities, and budgets must be prevented, and this is a responsibility of management. Automation in the hospital and in the physical therapy department can assist managerial and supervisory functions, but in the long run the effectiveness of these functions depends less on machines and gadgets than it does on management principles and style.

Management Style

Every manager makes assumptions about people, and these assumptions determine in large part how the manager deals with subordinates, peers, and superiors (24). Hickok's distinction between "defensive supervision" and "participative supervision" in physical therapy illustrates this point well (11).

Defensive supervision, based on high fear and low trust, is marked by close checks on hourly personnel, frequent reports, orders without explanations, strict rules, frequent inspections, withholding of information from subordinates, insistence that people stay in channels, and generally using line authority to keep a tight rein on people and their activities. Participative supervision, on the other hand, is based on high trust and low fear and is marked by opportunities for staff to share and cooperate in determining objectives, to innovate and explore, and to participate fully in departmental activities (11).

A manager's style can lead him into committing the "seven deadly sins," discussed fully by Marcus (17):

1. using snap judgment in the selection of employees, rather than selection techniques and interviews;
2. letting the eager beaver's job grow like topsy while letting the goldbrick get away with substandard performance;
3. failure to make assignments and instructions clear, in a courteous manner, and with enough authority to the people who are to carry them out;
4. being a boss instead of a leader;
5. being indifferent toward discipline and recognition when they are warranted;
6. being too busy to train subordinates, and instead applying pressure to increase productivity; and
7. playing everything close to the chest.

In contrast to the seven deadly sins, Hickok offers what we can call the "six virtues" of the effective supervisor (11):

1. has confidence in his or her ability to lead, and confidence in subordinates;
2. creates a climate of involvement for all staff members;
3. maintains open channels of communication in all directions and for all levels of staff members;
4. delegates responsibility with commensurate authority;
5. delineates clearly the assigned responsibility in keeping with the staff member's capacity to carry out the responsibility; and
6. offers staff members opportunities for professional growth.

The reader who studies the above sins and virtues carefully will recognize that they are based on underlying assumptions about people as employees and as managers or supervisors. The kinds of underlying assumptions that might be held, the managerial strategies they foster, and the implications for motivating employees are addressed in some detail later in this chapter.

Two implications of management style deserve consideration here. In advocating participative supervision in physical therapy, Hickok's final sentence is, "Today's effective supervisor must make decisions, provide leadership, and most important, *train the next generation of supervisors*" (11, emphasis added). By emphasizing staff involvement and participation, participative supervision quite naturally leads to a conclusion that the next generation of supervisors should be trained and that the method for doing this lies within the management style itself. Defensive supervision leads to no such conclusion. Good managerial talent is always in short supply, and its development cannot be left to learning by trial and error. Each hospital and each department should do two things. First, it needs to select the personnel with the greatest potential for managerial and supervisory positions, and, second, it ought to develop them to the point where they can fulfill their responsibilities and obligations to themselves, their profession, and the organization.

The second implication has to do with documented observations about national productivity. For many years, the United States was preeminent throughout the world for its productivity and for its development of managers and supervisors. More recently, Japan has been outstripping the United States in productivity, largely, the experts think, because of the management style and strategy adopted by Japanese industry where (a) emphasis is placed on communication and initiative from the bottom up in the pyramidal structure, (b) top management serves as a facilitator of decisions rather than as a source of edicts, (c) middle management serves as the impetus for and shaper of solutions to problems, (d) decisions are made by consensus, and (e) close attention is paid to the well-being of employees (23).

The evidence accumulating in the industrial and organizational psychology literature over the last 50 years indicates that the management style adopted by Japanese industry should be more effective than the old classical style of authority and hierarchy. Perhaps our industry has been too slow in breaking with tradition.

Manager as Leader

The fourth deadly sin mentioned earlier was "Being a boss instead of a leader." Ross offers some useful guidelines on what it takes for a manager to be an effective leader in an organization where the primary concern is productivity (23):

1. resolve conflicts early, with emphasis on the results expected of people.
2. allow participation in decision-making for the common good, not for good working relations.
3. encourage creativity and innovation.
4. manage by results, with emphasis on upward communication.
5. provide control and feedback, with emphasis on results expected, information on progress, and information for self-control.
6. maintain morale, with emphasis on good performance and opportunities, not problems.
7. negotiate and maintain a mutual commitment to goals.
8. use performance appraisal for setting future objectives, rather than for rewarding or punishing past performance based on judgement of traits (interest, enthusiasm, courtesy, etc.).
9. provide subordinates with opportunities for growth.
10. exert a positive impact on the organization's longevity and growth.

Ross also offers some advice on delegating to subordinates: delegate by results expected and match responsibility with authority; communicate: and maintain broad control by trusting the subordinates and expecting self-control (23).

MANAGEMENT FOR MOTIVATION

A primary responsibility of the manager or supervisor, and often a difficult one to fulfill, is motivating subordinates to take on the organization's goals as their own goals of work, the assumption being that this commitment will enhance productivity. The difficulty arises when the human element interjects a variable over which management has only limited control. In dealing with employees, the intangible factor of will, volition, or freedom of choice is introduced. Workers can increase or decrease their productivity as they choose.

Differences in management style and strategies may be based upon different assumptions about people, as mentioned in the previous section, but the different styles and strategies have a common purpose—getting subordinates to do what has to be done effectively and efficiently in order to achieve the organization's goals. Getting people to do something means motivating them. And motivating people can include a full spectrum of methods, from manipulation and coercion at one extreme, to people convincing themselves that they want to do what needs to be done.

Nature of Man

Historically, the assumptions about people in organizations—and the management styles based on those assumptions—have reflected different philosophical positions on the nature of man (the reader should know that "man" is used here and below in its generic sense to include both men and women). In recent years, theories of motivation have arisen from or have been related to these philosophical positions on the nature of man. These positions are used below as the key elements around which to present management styles and relevant theories of motivation. Much of what follows is taken from Schein (24), with other sources as noted.

Rational-Economic Man

Historically the oldest and longest enduring, the doctrine of rational-economic man holds that employees are motivated primarily by economic incentives and gain; that employees will rationally do whatever gets them the greatest economic gain; that employees' feelings are irrational and can interfere with their rational self-interest in economic gain; and, that employees can be manipulated, motivated by incentives, and controlled.

Some additional assumptions for this doctrine were later posed (but not advocated) by McGregor in what he called his Theory X (22): Employees lack initiative, they have natural or personal goals that run counter to those of the organization, and they are incapable of self-discipline and self-control.

The assumptions underlying the doctrine of rational-economic man quite naturally lead to the conclusion that management must motivate by manipulating economic incentives (reward and punishment), must control discipline and adherence to the organization's goals by managerial authority and force, and must achieve the motivation and control by planning and organizing.

Primary emphasis is on efficient task performance. Concern for the feelings and morale of employees is secondary. Problems of performance and productivity are solved by redesigning jobs and organizational relationships, or by changing the incentive and control systems. Under this doctrine, the burden of organizational performance falls upon management. Employees are expected to do no more than the incentive and control systems are designed to encourage and allow.

The management style that follows from this doctrine was quite successful in achieving industrialization and mass production. The classical pyramidal structure of organizations and line relationships (chain of command) probably have their roots in the doctrine of rational-economic man.

The assumptions underlying this doctrine and management style came into question as unions came into existence, as jobs became more complex, and as organizations had to rely more and more on their employees' judgment, creativity, and loyalty. Findings in industrial psychology also had their effect on the doctrine by showing that employees' needs affect productivity. The well-known Hawthorne studies (so-called from the plant in which they were conducted) demonstrated that employees have a need to be accepted and liked by their co-workers, that they resist being put into work situations which require competition with their co-workers, and that they work hard if they feel that management views their work as special, important, or new (19).

Social Man

The assumptions underlying the doctrine of social man, based chiefly on Mayo's findings in the Hawthorne studies (19), are that employees are motivated by social needs, that employees obtain their sense of identity and meaning of work through their social relationships at work, that employees are more responsive to the social forces of their peer group at work than they are to the incentives and controls of management, and that employees are responsive to management if management meets their social needs and their needs for acceptance.

The management style that follows from this doctrine is one in which the manager gives more attention to the needs of the employees and to their feelings of acceptance, belonging, and identity. Emphasis is placed on group incentives rather than individual incentives, and the manager's role shifts from one of planning, organizing, motivating, and controlling to one of serving as an intermediary between employees and higher management. The initiative for work—the source of motivation—shifts from management to employees. Through participative involvement, employees expect that some of their social needs will be met, and they become involved in and committed to the organization's goals.

Subsequent studies and theories, looking beyond social needs to the need to use capacities and skills in a mature and productive way, called into question the assumptions and the management style of the doctrine of social man.

Self-Actualizing Man

The doctrine of self-actualizing man differs from that of social man in one important premise: employees find meaning in work not so much through meeting their social needs as through achieving self-esteem, autonomy, and maximum use of their capacities and skills. The assumptions underlying this doctrine are based upon the work and ideas of Argyris (1), Herzberg (10), Maslow (18), McClelland (20), and McGregor—the latter's Theory Y, not Theory X mentioned in the discussion of rational-economic man (22).

1. Employees' motives are arranged in a hierarchy from lowest to highest: (a) needs for survival, safety, and security; (b) social needs; (c) needs for self-esteem; (d) needs for autonomy; and (e) needs for maximum use of all their resources (self-actualization).
2. Employees want to be mature on the job, to exercise a certain amount of independence, to develop special capacities and skills, and to achieve (to avoid failure).
3. Employees are primarily self-motivated and self-controlled.
4. Given the opportunity, employees will integrate their own goals with the organization's goals, that is, self-actualization poses no conflict with effective performance of the organization.

Job satisfaction is obviously closely related to several of the assumptions listed above. Herzberg's two-factor theory of job satisfaction is of special interest here (10). The theory holds that recognition, achievement, opportunity for advancement, responsibility, the possibility of growth, and work itself are "motivators" in the sense that they produce job satisfaction if they are present, but their absence does not necessarily produce job dissatisfaction. The theory also holds that working conditions, attributes of supervisors, salary, personnel policies, job security, status, and interpersonal relationships are "hygiene factors" in the sense that the negative aspects of these factors produce job dissatisfaction but their positive aspects do not necessarily produce job satisfaction. Just how all of this might apply to physical therapists in private practice and in practice as directors of departments can be found in the study reported by Barnes and Crutchfield (2). Examples of motivators and hygiene factors surrounding the job of staff secretary can be found in Ross (23).

The manager who holds to the doctrine of self-actualizing man will seek ways to make work more challenging and meaningful to employees; will serve as a catalyst and facilitator for employees satisfying their higher level needs; and will delegate responsibility and authority to subordinates, while at the same time giving up some of the traditional management prerogatives. Motivation shifts from being a trait to be stimulated to being one for which opportunities are to be provided. The notion of "growing in the job" has its base in this doctrine, as does the notion of enlarging the job to meet the employee's capabilities and skills. Ross makes the point that delegation of the manager's own duties is the best way to enlarge the job of subordinates (23).

Compared to the two doctrines discussed earlier, the one on self-actualizing man appears to apply as well as to managers and supervisors as it does to other employees. In fact, Schein suggests that the assumptions underlying this doctrine may be most relevant to managers, professionals, and other more highly educated employees because the evidence is not clear that employees at lower levels or with less education expect satisfaction of the higher level needs in their work (24). Schein goes on to suggest that the old adage of "a fair day's work for a fair day's pay" may be the principle expectation of employees who work to make enough money to find meaning and challenge *off* the job.

No one of the three doctrines on the nature of man can be generalized to all working men and women. Schein summarized the evidence in support of each; came to the conclusion that man is more complex than any of the three simplified doctrines: and proposed several assumptions for a fourth view, that of complex man (24).

Complex Man

Schein's assumptions about complex man, briefly summarized, are as follows (24):

1. Employees are complex, highly variable individuals who have motives arranged in some hierarchy of importance to them individually, and this hierarchy may change from time to time and from situation to situation.
2. Employees are capable of learning new motives and new patterns or combinations of motives through their organizational experiences.
3. Both formal and informal organizations may exist within a complex organization, and many jobs are complex in that they may require one employee to assume several roles. An employee's motives may vary among the different formal and informal organizations in which he is involved at work, as well as among the different roles he assumes.
4. Employees can become productively involved with an organization on the basis of many different motives. Job satisfaction and effective performance depend upon not only motivation but nature of the task, abilities and experience, and traits of co-workers.
5. Employees can respond differently to any one management style, just as they can respond effectively to different management styles. No one style or strategy will work for all employees all the time.

Another idea worth considering here is Vroom's conclusion that job performance and satisfaction is a function of the abilities the employee perceives to be required to do the job, the degree to which the employee thinks that he has those abilities, and the value the employee places on having those abilities (27).

The management style and strategy that follows from these assumptions about complex man requires that the manager be a good diagnostician of individual differences, be personally flexible, have a wide range of skills and knowledge, and place a high value on inquiry or problem-solving (1, 15, 22, 24). The successful manager must be sensitive to and value the differences among subordinates, and must know enough about the underlying assumptions and management styles of the three doctrines discussed earlier to be able to apply and test appropriate strategies and to change them as needed. The point is not to throw up one's hands in despair over the fact that people differ but to find out what management style works with whom and when.

Individual differences aside, the evidence is strong that employee participation in decision-making contributes importantly to productivity, job satisfaction, and growth in the job (24). The recent Japanese industrial experience, mentioned in the previous section, seems to offer some real world confirmation of the research findings in industrial psychology.

Personnel Motivation Problems in the Clinic

Many of management's problems with motivation of employees are based on an attempt to induce the worker to be more productive by offering rewards to be enjoyed off rather than on the job. A check of collective bargaining contracts in our field reveals this finding. Few hospitals and other health agencies try to make actual job performance a rewarding experience in itself. Very few routine jobs offer the rewards of achievement, recognition, work responsibility, and advancement. These rewards all too often must be obtained by employees spending their time at home working on projects they enjoy and for which they do the planning and make the decisions. If we as supervisors could take some of this enthusiasm and harness it to the job, considerable increase in productivity and job satisfaction could result.

There are, no doubt, situations in which an employee is blocked and frustrated at all attempts to get satisfaction from the job. This frustration is sometimes expressed in hostility, conflict, grievances, spoilage, destruction of property, and insubordination. Another manifestation of this frustration is the withdrawing in spirit from the job, a situation that is most disheartening for the supervisor. The worker refuses to use initiative or to participate in the work situation beyond just what is required. He may become indolent, passive, unwilling to accept responsibility, and even unreasonable in demands for wages, hours, vacations, holidays, and other economic benefits.

Every supervisor knows there are problem employees: those who are irresponsible, the troublemakers, the cry babies, the alcoholics, the long weekenders, the continuous vacationers, the health service buffs, etc. They exist in all segments of society, and health workers are not exempt. As a supervisor, be sure you can handle the situation before undertaking a solution. Seek guidance and direction from another department which might be better suited to handling the problem. I have found that the mental stress exhibited by some employees is usually caused by poor placement, insecurity, fear of being hurt, gripes, grievances, resentments, and frustrations. The supervisor can sometimes help a worker over a difficult time by changing the worker's job or by assigning the individual to a more congenial work group. The worker must know how far he can go with substandard performance and should be willing to talk to the supervisor or someone recommended by the supervisor. The supervisor should not take the responsibility for solving the subordinate's problems. He may point out solutions, but the person who has to live with the solution should have the opportunity to make the choice.

Summing-Up on Motivation

Any discussion of motivation must emphasize that each person is a unique being. Employees come to the work place a product of their home life, intellectual ability, and emotional makeup. Friends and families have affected their life styles. They are changed by experiences, education, and training. All things in life plus the situation of the moment enter into shaping their thinking about what they want out of life, how they will go about getting it, and how much effort they feel must be expended to get it. People do change. New experiences affect their way of perceiving. Supervisors would do well to recognize these ideas and realize that they cannot treat people alike. They must take individual differences into account in fitting people to jobs, in making assignments, in praising and rewarding, in criticizing, and in disciplining.

Physical therapist supervisors should consider what people want out of work. The assumptions, theories, and management styles discussed above provide a comprehensive source of factors to consider. Another source is Herzberg's review of research on what people want out of work (9). Herzberg compiled the following list, in order of preference, from surveys of people who were employed, out of work, applying for work, and quitting:

1. security,
2. work that is meaningful,
3. opportunity for advancement,
4. recognition,
5. competent leadership,
6. fair wages,
7. freedom from arbitrary action,
8. a voice in matters affecting them,
9. congenial associates, and
10. satisfactory working conditions.

Finally, managers and supervisors who have themselves and their jobs under control are usually calm, friendly, and understanding and can do much to alleviate any tension that may exist. Their style of conduct and how they deal with others sets up a work climate that is either harmonious or full of stress. Their concern for seeing that things go well can provide an environment in which subordinates do get pleasure from each day's work.

COMMUNICATION

As used in this chapter, communication means the *interchange* of information, ideas, and feelings. Used in this way, communication includes sending, receiving, understanding, and responding to messages that may be conveyed in oral or written form, by actions, and by body language (gestures, postures, and facial expressions). By using the word communication to refer to the interchange of the content of messages, we can avoid careless uses of the word—as in, "I sent him three communications (actually, three memos) last week"—and we can come closer to what communication is all about in personnel management.

The previous discussions of management, supervision and management for motivation show quite clearly that communication in the form of interchange of information, ideas, and feelings is absolutely necessary, a *sine qua non*, for effective management and supervision of personnel. This notion is supported by Brennan, who states that an organization, whatever its size or mission, functions through its people, who in turn function through communication, and that, in effect, communication is the glue that holds an organization together (4).

To some people, ours is the age of communication. That impression may exist because of the bombardment by the media, the instantaneous coverage of events anywhere in the world, and the explosion of technology in the electronics industry. Perhaps the age is one of communication problems created not only by the bombardment of messages but also by the increasing size and complexity of our organizations. Technological advances can assist communication in hospitals and other health care settings, but Brown cautions that technical communication devices can divert attention away from the fact that communication is more a matter of minds than of machines (5).

This section of the chapter addresses the structure and climate for effective communication and the manager or supervisor as a sender and as a listener.

The fact that organizations continue to adhere to the classical pyramidal structure and hierarchical lines of authority (for a number of good reasons) places the burden upon managers and supervisors at all levels to establish and maintain an effective communication climate in spite of the prevailing structure. Brennan has summarized the principal characteristics of a health communication climate as being those that (4):

1. enable people to form positive relationships;
2. allow people to participate in the communication process;
3. permit people to believe much of what they hear from managers and supervisors;
4. bring people in frequent contact with those who influence their economic and emotional rewards; and

5. foster a sense of satisfaction through dialogue, participating, contributing, and the feeling of belonging.

To foster effective communication, management at all levels must value the free flow of information and establish an atmosphere in which truth and openness prevail. A relationship of trust between employees and supervisors at all levels helps to overcome the human failings that cause people to "color" information as it is passed along. It takes courage at times for subordinates to tell their superiors the truth. If telling the truth is met with varying degrees of displeasure, employees soon learn to doctor the information to suit the particular superior's taste. Information can be selected, doubtful situations discussed optimistically, and bad news withheld. One soon learns what must be done in place of a relationship of trust, integrity, and understanding.

Where a supervisor encourages mutual liking and trust, subordinates know that they can question and be listened to in a way that will result in understanding. Nothing deters the formulation and implementation of ideas more than a lack of understanding, trust, and respect between the supervisor and his staff.

An important determiner of success for anyone as supervisor is the objective of developing attitudes that facilitate understanding. A supervisor who takes the time and allows subordinates to develop positive attitudes about him, will find that they will work with him in achieving goals. He must demonstrate a willingness to be concerned about their welfare, an understanding of their problems, and an appreciation of them as individuals. It has been demonstrated many times that the better the relationships a supervisor has with his subordinates, the more they will help him in his job of communicating with them. Also, if the supervisor has taken the time to get to know his employees as individuals, to know their good points, their shortcomings, and their need for reassurance, warmth, and importance, they will realize that his feeling grumpy at times will not affect them adversely. The subordinates who feel secure in their relationships with the supervisor, who respect and trust him, will not misunderstand or misinterpret his intentions if he seems occasionally cross or abrupt. Without this feeling of security, subordinates can become resentful, uncertain, and afraid to ask questions or make suggestions. And, of course, what has been said here about the male supervisor applies equally well to the female supervisor.

The staff conference can be a useful means of helping to establish an effective communication climate, but not if the conference is held infrequently, limited to senior-level staff, or run in a perfunctory manner (5). A memorandum from the "busy" manager or supervisor is not an adequate substitute for a meeting. Limiting staff conferences to senior level or upper level staff members provides a clear message to others that they are unimportant. And any meeting in which subordinates sit around for the sole purpose of accepting what a superior puts before them has a deadening effect on the communication climate.

A poor or unsatisfactory communication climate fosters the development of informal, alternative communication networks that may be detrimental to the organization. Every organization has informal communication networks, often among employees of similar pay or responsibility levels. Thank goodness they do, because these informal networks probably help employees meet their social needs at work. Informal networks that may be detrimental are grapevines and their sources of information, the rumor mills.

Rumors tend to be most rampant in those departments where the supervisors deliberately withhold information. Once fed into the grapevine, the rumor spreads faster than any official message through official channels because the grapevine is informal and the rumor is usually "hot news." It is said that almost anyone who is confused or doubtful about what is going on becomes the more active user of this kind of communication, and in any organization this can include all employees who feel that they are shut out of participating in decisions that affect them.

The grapevine is an unreliable, and sometimes inaccurate, means of communication. Because it can do irreparable damage to a work group or to an individual, managers and supervisors should apply their best efforts to prevent rumors and minimize the effects of the grapevine. The old adage, "An ounce of prevention is worth a pound of cure," applies here. Establish a climate of trust, honesty, openness, and understanding. If rumors circulate, analyze their frequency and type. This analysis can be helpful. It may indicate where in the structure the formal communication network is not being allowed to function, and it may show areas of employee interest, of poor morale, and of misinformation or missing information.

Manager or Supervisor as Sender

The physical therapist manager or supervisor sends messages every day, and often throughout the day, to subordinates. This conveying of messages occurs every time the manager or supervisor:

1. delegates responsibility and authority;
2. makes assignments and changes in assignments;
3. gives directions, advice and counsel;
4. answers questions and responds to complaints;
5. praises and reprimands; and
6. interprets and enforces policies and regulations.

The message conveyed in each case depends not only on the verbal (oral or written) content but also on how the message is conveyed. Style, tone, clarity, and organization of presentation are essential for conveying the intended oral or written message. Brown refers to these requirements as "the precise and demanding art of translating concepts into words, sentences, and paragraphs" (5). Of course, meeting these requirements does not assure that the message will be understood. Many factors can interfere with a message being understood, and not all of these factors are under the control of the manager or supervisor. Style, tone, clarity, and organization of the supervisor's messages are, however, under his or her control, and failure to meet these requirements will contribute to the message not being understood.

Facial expressions, hand and shoulder gestures, and body postures markedly influence how the content of the oral message is conveyed. This body language can enhance the intended meaning of the message, or it can distract from or totally distort the intended meaning. Consider the subordinate who seeks a decision from a supervisor and is told, in reply, "I think you should make that decision." With one set of facial expressions and gestures, this reply would mean, "I have confidence in your ability to make a sound decision. Go ahead. I trust you." With a different set of facial expressions and gestures, this reply could mean, "Why are you bothering me with this matter? Get off my back. Go make the decision yourself, like you're supposed to do." A deadpan expression and no gestures could leave the receiver not knowing what the *real* meaning of the message was.

Three important points follow from the considerations posed above: (a) the personality of the sender is part of the message, especially in areas concerned with standards, values, purposes, and motivation (5); (b) a good manager or supervisor takes the approach of a teacher in conveying messages, being more concerned with understanding than with passive acceptance (5); and (c) whenever possible, written messages should be followed with oral messages to help enhance understanding.

In spite of the care taken in preparing the presentation of a message, the manager or supervisor should not be surprised if part of the message fails to get through, or gets through and is forgotten, or gets through but is misunderstood. Borrowing from the approach of a teacher can help: do appropriate checks at periodic intervals, clarify by citing examples, and periodically review the content by repeating it in different ways. Supervisors also soon learn that a message requiring action will be carried out more intelligently and more willingly if the subordinate knows why he or she was chosen to do it, how important it is, and what will be done with the information. Most people want to know that what they do is important. This not only becomes a way of communicating intelligently, but may also enhance any schemes for motivating employees.

What has been said about conveying messages to subordinates applies equally well to conveying messages to would-be subordinates (job applicants) and to superiors. In both of these instances, the manager or supervisor will usually go to greater pains to make certain that the messages are clear, logically organized, and persuasive—especially if the applicant is a desirable candidate for a vacant position or if the message to the superior is a proposed increase in the budget. The responsibility to convey messages to subordinates should receive the same care and be undertaken with the same enthusiasm.

Recruitment of personnel is considered later in this chapter. The responsibilities of the manager or supervisor in communicating with superiors are many and important, but a full discussion of these responsibilities falls outside the scope of this chapter on personnel management.

Manager or Supervisor as Listener

Epictetus, a Greek philosopher, suggested in his *Discourses* that "Nature has given men one tongue, but two ears, that we may hear from others twice as much as we speak." If listening and speaking really worked this way, there would be nothing to say in this section.

Brennan makes a useful distinction between "management by mouth" and "management by ear" (4). Management by mouth is characterized by the manager or supervisor who dominates every discussion with subordinates, tells people what to do instead of asking for opinions about how to do the job better, threatens rather than encourages, and generally treats employees as adolescents. Management by ear, on the other hand, is characterized by the manager or supervisor who not only talks with but listens to employees, is interested in their views, solicits their suggestions and opinions, is sensitive to their aspirations and needs, and communicates with rather than at them.

Learning how to listen with the ears open and the mouth closed is a prerequisite to communicating effectively in any situation. Being a good listener requires that one learn how to interpret the spoken word in light of facial and bodily signs. A supervisor soon realizes how important it is to be a good listener and to be approachable and friendly so that subordinates will come forward with questions and comments about things that might be puzzling to them. The supervisor has to learn to ask questions in a manner that inspires trust and helps to draw out information and opinion. The skilled supervisor sifts through feedback bit by bit so that the give and take of a discussion truly goes in at least two directions. To be accused of a one-way discussion changes the meaning of discussion with overtones of autocracy; soon the supervisor loses all possibility of conversation with the staff. It is well-known that accuracy and comprehension increase with the amount of feedback in conversation.

Effective listening is a skill to be learned through practice. Some keys to effective listening are (6):

1. Listen for ideas or major themes, rather than facts.
2. Judge the content, not the delivery; that is, put the burden on yourself as a listener rather than on the person who is speaking.
3. Don't respond to "trigger" words by leaping in before the speaker finishes.
4. Work at listening. Thought is faster than speech. Use listening time to review, evaluate, and summarize what the speaker has said.
5. Resist distractions.

By way of summary, being an effective listener requires overlooking in other speakers some of the flaws that one should avoid in one's own presentation of messages. The manager or supervisor who works at being an effective listener and an effective presenter will contribute much to the communication climate and may even reach a point of being able to help subordinates learn these skills.

RECRUITMENT AND SELECTION

The purpose of recruitment and selection is to fill positions with the best candidates from among persons who are qualified for those positions. By "best candidates" I mean those persons whose abilities, backgrounds, personalities, interests, ambitions, and goals indicate that they (a) are best suited for the specifications and duties of the jobs, (b) will contribute most to achieving the department's goals and objectives, and (c) demonstrate the greatest potential for growth.

Recruitment

In its simplest form, recruitment means attracting applicants from outside the organization. Recruitment may be passive for positions at some levels, or for some facilities, if applicants are already attracted by the possibility of employment (e.g., as physical therapy aides, or possibly as clerical or secretarial help) or by the reputation, program, or location of the facility (as is sometimes the case with physical therapist and physical therapist assistant applicants).

Active recruitment consists of advertising in professional journals, newsletters, and newspapers; contacting physical therapist and physical therapist assistant educational programs, or participating in their clinical education affiliation programs, or visiting their campuses to actively recruit, or any combination of these methods; participating in placement service activities or recruiting informally at professional conferences and meetings; and using the services of external employment and placement services. Active recruitment implies offering lures to attract applicants. The lures may be financial, intellectual, and even recreational. Consider a few examples of lures offered recently to physical therapists:

"Fringe benefits: paid health plan, paid vacation, paid sick leave, 11 paid holidays, 5 paid personal days, as well as a New York State employee's pension plan."

"Opportunity—To live, work, and enjoy fantastic outdoor recreational activities in the Rocky Mountains."

"Unique Opportunities—For professional and personal development of physical therapist with master's degree...clinical specialization in care of patients with spinal cord injury, brain injury, or amputation; administration. Research program directed by...; education program (staff development, fellowship program for new graduates with master's degree, continuing education) directed by...."

And here's one for the physical therapist assistant:

"Expanding acute/skilled care facility in a charming small town with a colonial heritage.... Enjoy the beautiful beaches of the Outer Banks."

Aggressive recruitment is going after particular individuals because of their known expertise and reputation. To attract such individuals away from their current work and home settings may require offering specific high level responsibilities and opportunities, relocation expenses, laboratory space, and other prerequisites peculiar to the position.

In sheer numbers, most recruitment efforts are directed toward attracting applicants for staff physical therapist positions. And most of these efforts are what I call active recruitment. In the early 1970s, when the first edition of this book was prepared, there appeared to be a slight surplus of physical therapists in some parts of the country. The impression then was that recruitment might become more passive and that increasing emphasis could be placed on selection, that is, being selective in selection. Now, by the 1980s, the tide seems to have turned. The demand for physical therapists is high, and active recruitment seems to be at an all-time high. This scenario suggests an interesting relationship between recruitment and selection.

When the number of potential applicants exceeds the demand for a particular level of personnel, recruitment can be essentially passive (except, perhaps, for the remote or relatively unknown facility) and selection becomes a high intensity activity. When, however, the demand for a particular level of personnel exceeds the number of potential applicants, recruitment becomes a high intensity activity and selection may "atrophy" from disuse. Under the latter condition, which is upon us now, the search becomes one of finding the warm bodies with the minimal qualifications to fill the positions. This sorry state of affairs does not bode well for the future development of the main core of our profession. All is not bleak, however.

The advertised "positions available" in 1980 are not only more numerous than they were almost a decade ago but are also more specific in terms of special clinical programs in existence or planned and in terms of special experience desired in applicants. The trend toward specialized programs and practice and toward clinical research is providing both potential applicants and employers areas of concentration within which both recruitment and selection can be more selective.

Aggressive recruitment (also called "robbing" other facilities) to fill top level clinical positions in physical therapy is just getting under way and will probably increase as hospitals and other health care settings pursue opportunities for special programs and clinical research. Search committees to identify top flight talent in the field, long a practice in academic settings, is becoming a practice in health care settings. This trend may affect the long held tradition in many facilities of making promotions to top level positions from within the organization. Promotion from within provides opportunities for staff development (and motivation) and it gives the employer the advantage of known performance, but it may not bring to the organization the special talents and experiences it needs for developing in new directions.

Job Specifications and Duties

Actually, before recruitment of applicants for a position begins—and certainly before a selection is made—the specifications and duties for the job should be determined. As a general rule, the job specifications and duties for lower level positions are determined in advance and are somewhat less flexible than those for higher level positions. The job specifications and duties for a higher level position may be developed and changed in the course of talking with prospective applicants, and especially in matching the job with the personal characteristics of the most likely candidate. While the job specifications and duties of any position may change as an employee grows in the job, it is unlikely that those of a lower level position will change in the course of interviewing prospective applicants.

Feitelberg presents 13 categories of job specifications that are applicable to positions at all levels in the typical physical therapy department (7). A few examples will suffice here: minimum education requirements, specialized or advanced education requirements, required experience, physical demands, internal and external relationships, promotion opportunities, and salary or wage scale.

The job duties describe what the person in the position is to do and how the duties are to be accomplished. The job specifications and job duties, along with job title, name and title of immediate superior, and job summary, make up the job description. A full discussion of purposes, format, uses, and development of job descriptions can be found in Feitelberg (7).

Selection

The selection function of any organization constitutes one of the most important supervisory responsibilities.

I have for many years considered as two of my major responsibilities, as a supervisor and a director of a physical therapy department, the proper selection and development of staff. The latter is discussed later in this chapter.

I have adhered to a certain philosophy in selecting physical therapists and other staff members. The comments that follow reflect my selection philosophy.

We need men and women of talent whose mental ability, creativity, and initiative will continue to lead our profession and our organizations along the path of success.

This kind of personnel is needed at all levels where the capacity for independent actions can spell the difference between success or failure of the organization to deliver its service and of the individual to contribute. No matter what incursions are made by the bugaboo of automation, remember that it is people who are still needed to run our business and our departments, and to treat our patients. The future of our particular brand of health care delivery depends upon these employees, upon the work they have been trained to perform, and upon the ideas that they contribute toward improvement in our delivery system. The supervisor, the manager, or the administrator has as a main function the task of assembling individuals into a productive, dynamic, harmonious work group. The importance to the individual of proper selection and placement is also of prime concern. His own goals, motives, and objectives must be realized by this cooperative effort.

A work force, at all levels, is a dynamic group in constant action and reaction. It must, by necessity, be composed of members who come to the department with unique personalities. A supervisor must early recognize the fact that the only way to strengthen the group and to keep it dynamic is to attempt continually to improve the caliber of the people selected for the various positions. The selective hiring of a sufficient number of qualified individuals is significant in that they furnish the source for present and future talent in the organization and in the profession.

As each person is selected for his specific job, the selection process must include those who have potential for supervising, managing, teaching, or research. If the prospective employee has other plans, you may not be able to set the stage for his development. This should be ascertained at the intake interview. Nevertheless, the basic philosophy of growth should in all cases be aimed at developing the person's best possible potential.

All supervisors must select personnel with the future uppermost in mind. People must be made to think of what they would like to be doing one, three, or five years hence and be given to realize how important this projected thinking is for themselves and for the organization.

The selection procedure, to be most effective, must match the personal characteristics of the potential employee with the requirements of the specific position available. Much care should be used in matching personal abilities with job requirements. The certificate or diploma, for example, should not be considered the sole basis for selection. One of the disadvantages of this source is the high rate of turnover seen in new graduates. Experience in this regard suggests that many new graduates will stay approximately two to three years and will move on to better paying jobs, graduate schools, marriage and family, or different geographical locations. This comment is made not to denigrate new graduates but only to illustrate one of the problems of the "warm body" approach to selecting personnel.

The matching procedure begins with an awareness of and evaluation of all known assets and liabilities of the employee. It is not only an injustice to place a person on a job that demands less ability than he has but, more importantly, it is a source of employee dissatisfaction, loss of initiative, and most probably loss to the organization of the person. One prevailing assumption is that more able persons should not do work that less able persons can do. Another view holds that the "proper use" of a person's capabilities requires a balance between peak demands and normal use; that is, there should be some routine tasks to execute along with the more difficult problems that challenge the person's ability.

The comments offered above represent a philosophy that can be applied to full information on applicants and a full description of job specifications and duties in making a selection. The alternative, which is not yet available in physical therapy, is a scientific approach to establishing predictor variables to be used in selection (24, pp. 18–26). Interestingly, the two approaches look at the same kinds of information on applicants:

1. biographical information and work history;
2. intellectual level and aptitude;
3. specific areas of knowledge and specific skills;
4. attitudes and interests; and
5. motivation, personality, and temperament.

Every supervisor wants to select employees who will be successful on the job. Success on the job is often determined by three things (14):

1. intellectual and physical capability;
2. education, training, and experience; and
3. motivation to succeed.

In many cases ambition and ability may be far more meaningful to success than a formal education (12).

Other success indicators in the matching process might be imagination, logic, insight into human nature, communication ability, and willingness to become involved in problem solving.

Additional Comments

The issues of manpower supply and the need and types of manpower needed ultimately affect the physical therapist manager's or supervisor's role and effectiveness in personnel management. These issues have shown themselves to be intractable, however, even in more closely studied health professions such as medicine and nursing. For example, a surplus of physicians has been predicted and may, in fact, occur; but the question of whether this is good or bad, or what the implications will be, has produced more heat than light. The controversy rages as this book goes to press.

The individual physical therapist manager or supervisor, in the meantime, must adopt a philosophy on recruitment and selection that takes into account the personnel needs in his own setting, the goals and objectives of the department, his own personal goals in assembling a staff, and the kinds of people he wishes to work with day in and day out.

One final note, visibility in the profession helps to attract applicants. Whatever the supply of potential applicants, the work, accomplishments, publications, and professional presentations of the existing staff—including the manager or supervisor—can go a long way in attracting staff who have the same aspirations.

PERFORMANCE APPRAISAL

Day after day the supervisor observes and appraises the performance of subordinates. The results of this ongoing appraisal should be shared with the individual staff members in the form of ongoing feedback. Praise, gratitude, constructive criticism, and correction are effective reinforcers if they are given at the time the performance is observed. Of course, any negative reinforcement should not be given "in public," that is, in front of patients, co-workers, or students. The point here is not to leave subordinates hanging in mid-air, so to speak, over how they are doing. Do not wait until the first formal appraisal to tell a subordinate what he should have done three months ago. Nobody likes surprises.

The ongoing performance appraisal described above is useful in two additional ways: (a) it serves as the basis for day-to-day decisions in assigning responsibilities, tasks, and patients; and, even more importantly for this section of the chapter, (b) it provides the documentable evidence needed at the time of the periodic, formal performance appraisal.

Periodic Appraisal

Most organizations require that periodic, formal (written) performance appraisals be made of all employees, and that these written appraisals be part of the organization's employee records. These periodic appraisals are commonly used to substantiate recommendations for salary increases, promotions, and, if need be, demotions and terminations.

As written records, the results of periodic appraisals are important to each employee, as part of his employment record for future reference, and to the organization, as substantiation for decisions made about employees. Because of the possibility that such records may be used as exhibits in legal proceedings or labor disagreements, the supervisor should set up some system of recording and data collection that can help in the appraisal period. Once a month reporting from which a 12-month document can be prepared brings to light facts and does away with the possibility of conjecture. It is essential that accurate and comprehensive records be kept on each member of the staff.

If an employee's work and behavior are so unsatisfactory that discharge is being considered, it is the evidence collected and recorded which gives support and credence to the final decision. Such documentation is equally important to support recommendations not to grant merit increases in salary, recommendations not to promote, and even recommendations to promote which may not be approved higher up in the organization and which later may be contested.

These comments about the importance of performance appraisals as records are meant to emphasize the care, seriousness, and fairness with which they need to be prepared. In some facilities, these appraisals are treated perfunctorily. Nobody benefits from that, including the employees.

Each employee has a right to periodic performance appraisals and to rational decisions, based on appraisal, about his job status, responsibilities, and salary. Without appraisal, a subordinate cannot know what kind of performance a superior expects or considers important.

The relationship between the supervisor and the subordinate which was begun at the induction interview continues during subsequent appraisal periods. The appraisal process is the means by which the supervisor tells the employee how he is doing. The process should be used as a stimulant to continued learning and growth on the job, so that the employee can be ready by experience and other requirements for the advancements that should be available. If the employee is not doing well, he is entitled to a warning and to counseling on what potentially is wrong and what should be done to correct it. If he is not suited to the full extent of the job, he must find this out before investing too much time in it and so have the chance to seek other opportunities.

Many organizations use their own standardized forms to appraise performance, behavior, abilities, and potential. Formal appraisal should occur at regular intervals, should be done by the immediate supervisor, and should be made known to each employee. The appraisal interview and discussion with the employee should be completed by the immediate supervisor; it should be part of a program with promotability and should concentrate on improving the effectiveness of performance on the present job; it should also be a means of increasing the effectiveness of performance. In spite of some negative connotations, feedback on employee performance is vital to an effective supervisor-employee relationship. The majority of professional and support staff for whom appraisal becomes a regular occurrence find it a useful and rewarding experience.

In commenting upon the negative connotations of performance appraisal, Ross claimed that the typical emphasis on reward and punishment detracts from what the purpose should be—the setting of future personal objectives expressed in terms of results, and that any focus on personality traits is "bad news" for everybody, employee and supervisor alike (23). From a viewpoint of productivity as primary concern of any organization, Ross advocated that performance appraisal should focus on results rather than on activities and responsibilities. He sees the latter as a problem engendered by job descriptions, which typically address duties and responsibilities rather than expected results. These ideas are certainly worth considering as our field expands its attention to measuring outcomes.

Systematic, Unbiased Appraisal

Having to do a performance appraisal periodically, to put the results in writing, and to discuss the appraisal with the employee helps a great deal in making the appraisal systematic; that is, every employee can expect to go through the process periodically on a known date. The date might be, for example, each employee's anniversary date with the organization, or at the time of rotation from one unit to another within the department, or on a date that coincides in some way with the organization's fiscal year. Another suggestion along this line is to have the employee sign the written appraisal, not as an indication of his acceptance or approval but as evidence that a copy was shared at the time of the appraisal interview.

For a performance appraisal to be systematic, all employees holding positions at the same level (e.g., all staff physical therapists or all physical therapist assistants) should be judged on the same set of variables or factors. This, along with convenience, explains why rating forms are so often used in performance appraisals. Open-ended, narrative style written appraisals present a problem in this regard.

Systematic appraisal contributes to but does not assure an unbiased appraisal. An unbiased appraisal is one that is close to the truth, or as free of error as possible. Error occurs in an appraisal for a number of reasons, only some of which may actually be related to a supervisor's prejudice for or against certain persons on staff. For reasons of their own, some supervisors may routinely rate all performance too high or too low. As an appraiser, a good supervisor must be discriminating but not discriminatory, and not given to maternal or paternal instincts or to protecting one's own hide. Being unwilling, for any reason, to assign unfavorable ratings, favorable ratings, or extreme ratings in either direction will introduce error or bias into the appraisal. So, too, will being unwilling, or having neglected, to do the necessary work of appraisal—superficial impressions based upon insufficient observation are likely to be in error.

Rating forms and scales have many advantages, but if they are poorly prepared or designed they can make the appraisal vulnerable to error. Inadequate operational definitions for the factors to be rated, or factors that are not observable (e.g., potential, interest, attitude toward work), leave the way open for error or bias, as will any vagueness or ambiguity. Error will get into the appraisal if the categories on a rating scale are not mutually exclusive, that is, if the categories are defined in such a way that the person being rated can be placed in *either one* of *two* categories. Consider the following item on quantity of work, taken from an actual employee rating form:

Quantity
a.( ) Unusually high output—meets emergency demands well.
b.( ) Consistently turns out more than average.
c.( ) Finishes allotted amount.
d.( ) Does just enough to get by.
e.( ) Amount of work done is inadequate.

What of the employee who shows unusually high output but does *not* meet emergency demands well? Or, the employee who satisfies category b or c *and* meets emergency demands well? The dilemma usually arises when one or more of the categories on a scale are defined by a combination of two or more factors or variables. Employee rating forms and student rating forms commonly show this problem.

Error can also be introduced through the design of the rating form. Having a middle category on a scale (a scale with an odd number of categories) makes it easier for the rater to pick the middle if he is reluctant to assign extreme ratings or has not observed enough of the performance factor to make a decision. Having the category "Excellent" at the same end of the scale on every item in a rating form can produce the so-called "Halo effect," in which the rater is unduly influenced by a single favorable factor that influences the rating of all other factors. Actually, the Halo effect works either way—favorably or unfavorably. The name of the effect remains the same, and error is introduced either way.

Error or bias can also be reduced by training the supervisors as raters. The training or orientation should include explanation of the purpose of the rating form, information of the kind presented in this section of the chapter, and clarification of the meaning of the factors to be rated and the categories on the scales used for rating. Training sessions of this kind should be repeated periodically, and may even lead to improvements in the rating forms used in the facility. A member of the facility's personnel department may be called upon to assist with these training sessions.

To protect against prejudice and errors in judgment, some departments have more than one person share in the rating of an individual. A number of people who are acquainted with the worker and his work may act as a committee in making an appraisal. The employees should have a way of appealing the ratings if they consider them to be unfair. This point is now being built into collective bargaining contracts to minimize the possibility of unfairness. And, again, all ratings and comments in a performance appraisal should be based upon documented evidence.

Content of Appraisal

The factors or variables to be judged in a performance appraisal will vary with the level and type of positions held by employees. In any case, the manager or supervisor, or the organization itself, will determine what kinds of factors are most important in an appraisal.

I have found the following list of questions to be a useful guide in appraising the performance of employees and in letting them know the kinds of things that would be judged (and, of course, I urge the reader to seriously consider these questions as suggestions, and to overlook the repetitive use of the masculine gender—please consider "he," "his," and "him" to include "she" and "her"):

1. How well does he get along with others in the performance of his work?
2. Is he regular, steady, continually interested, and willing?
3. Does he need help and of what sort?

4. How does he comply with instructions, rules, policies, and department regulations?
5. Is safety for himself and others paramount in his thinking?
6. How much prodding if any does he need to get going on a project or on his schedule?
7. What sort of supervision is needed, if any?
8. Is he where he is supposed to be at the time he is supposed to be there?
9. What are his follow-through responsibilities and how are they done?
10. How does he use his initiative and creativity in improving his methods of care?
11. How flexible is he, and how adaptable is he to new and different thrusts and to changing ways?
12. Is he willing to involve himself in continuing education and to apply this new knowledge?
13. What are his potentials for promotion?
14. Does his expertise and competence allow him to be considered immediately for promotion? Do his co-workers and peers recognize this?

Alternative suggestions, applicable to physical therapist employees, can be found in Lister's article on using tasks and standards (16) and in McDaniel's article on the critical incident method (21). The interested reader may also find Wood's article on merit rating in physical therapy of help (28).

Appraisal Interview

Everything that has been said and suggested up to this point—and I do mean *everything*, not just performance appraisal—comes to bear upon the appraisal interview. The anticipation and the occasion of this interview can be discomforting for the superior as well as for the subordinate. This would-be supervisor, the relatively inexperienced supervisor, and the experienced supervisor who still dreads this "moment of truth" should read Wood's excellent review and discussion of the pros and cons of the appraisal interview (28). The comments and suggestions that follow reflect my experiences in using this type of interview.

It is the appraisal, a face-to-face communication between supervisor and subordinate, that can help the employee toward better performance, transfer to another job, or promotion to a higher level. All evidence on attitude, performance, absences, lateness, and quality and quantity of work should be on hand and should have been studied before the interview. A quiet time and place should be selected. It is important that a relaxed atmosphere be established and that the supervisor set the tone by accepting the fact that he must listen as well as share information.

Assuming that most performance appraisals reveal some area in need of improvement or further growth, subordinates should be encouraged to discuss openly their performance or any factors which make their jobs difficult.

Answers can come if subordinates are allowed to find their own solutions by simply opening their thought processes to patient, careful suggestion. Employees seem to be able to accept correction that relates to performance but not to their personalities. It is suggested that *no* criticism be even hinted at regarding personality. This kind of conversation becomes irrelevant and leads nowhere. Attempt to speak with employees, not at them or down to them. Let them know that you do care, identify specific areas which require improvement, and give suggestions and offer training recommendations regarding these areas.

The employee should be encouraged to work out a plan for improving performance with a definite schedule set up for it. My experience has been that when a time period for improvement is suggested, the employee gets started and can keep going to achieve the goal which has been set. Most people can be directed positively; therefore, the supervisor should also make arrangements for follow-up at specified times to see how improvement is going. The interested reader might wish to examine Zimmerman's example of an interview concerning tardiness (30).

At some time or another, every supervisor must come to grips with the dilemma of an unsatisfactory performer. We know that people who select a career in health are exceptional people. Nevertheless, the occasional unsatisfactory performer slips in. The supervisor should have clearly set in mind what action the interview should produce. All information to support the action should be in hand. The unsatisfactory rating must be justified and corrective action discussed with the worker. A timetable should be established which shows the required amount of improvement. It is essential to take written minutes which employee and supervisor both review. If, after the set time period improvement has not been demonstrated, then it becomes necessary to institute separation from the organization. This separation is more often a kindness than not. Much too often a supervisor procrastinates and allows an unsatisfactory performer to swing against the tide for a year or more. Be assured that the problem worsens and the whole department will soon react to this unsavory worker in its midst. Beware of such people and be aware of such procrastinating behavior on your part which will undermine all your other best efforts.

The supervisor must be able to use an interview style that suits his personality, that of the subordinate, and the circumstances of the situation. How can you handle the subordinate who disagrees with the performance evaluation? A suggestion that has been found acceptable is to ask the subordinate to evaluate his own performance. A comparison and discussion of each point must follow and the supervisor must keep the discussion on a plane where help can be given and help can be accepted by the subordinate. If an employee becomes angry, he should be encouraged to ventilate this anger. Whatever the reaction, the supervisor who has been fair, just, and honest makes every attempt to avoid argument. Arguing with an angry subordinate does not lead to a proper plan for future development. The supervisor's only concern should be to help the employee see the quality of his performance and how this may be assisted by suggestions for development and self-improvement. A close look at reality is called for before self-improvement can be obtained.

Generally, most employees will react positively to criticism that they see as constructive. It must be presented in a positive manner, however, and the employee will soon recognize that it is to his benefit to give it a positive reaction. Be wary of the employee who reacts negatively by blaming others, the workplace, policy, etc., while not seeing at all that his own self and attitudes may be at fault. You may not be able to help this person.

Appraisal of the Manager or Supervisor

The manager or supervisor also needs continued feedback, guidance, and support. He should also be evaluated on performance and potential for advancement to higher management jobs. His strongest personal characteristics and the areas in which he excels become important indicators of the direction of development. Just as he demonstrates an awareness of subordinates' needs, so his needs ought to be evaluated and met. He should be encouraged to build on strengths and should have help in improving weaknesses, much as is done for subordinates.

Unfortunately, the manager or supervisor rarely gets an explicit appraisal followed by an appraisal interview. The higher one goes in the management hierarchy, the more likely it is that an increase in salary, or a shifting of responsibilities, or a request for resignation becomes the chief form of appraisal and feedback.

A recent article by Fritz on self-assessment for the manager, while not 100 percent germane to the physical therapist manager or supervisor in a clinical facility, provides a comprehensive outline of factors to be judged in management style, planning, information/communication, time management, and delegation (8). The article provides a sound base for developing an appropriate managerial or supervisory appraisal in physical therapy.

RETENTION AND DEVELOPMENT

The concerns of the physical therapist manager or supervisor for staff retention and staff development reflect the dual role of this position. As an agent of higher management, the supervisor must be concerned with keeping enough competent employees for long enough periods of time to assure a reasonable degree of effectiveness and efficiency in carrying out the department's work and achieving its goals. Faced with a tight labor market and competition from other settings, the manager or supervisor may find retention, like recruitment, high on his list of priorities.

Ideally, the hospital or other health care facility should be committed to staff development, and the manager or supervisor should be obliged to implement this commitment in his role as an agent of higher management. Usually, however, the commitment arises from the supervisor's intent to help subordinates satisfy their higher level needs (see the earlier discussion in self-actualizing man), from his desire to enhance the quality of care provided in the department, and from his dedication to furthering the development of the field or profession in general. A deliberate, planned effort to improve, increase, and broaden the knowledge and skills of staff will produce benefits both within and outside the walls of the organization.

Staff development is an investment in people. Those who stay with the organization provide a direct return on this investment. Those who leave take the investment with them, but this does not necessarily represent an absolute loss to the organization. Indirect returns may come in the form of spreading reputation, attracting high caliber applicants and student affiliations, stimulating referrals, and so forth.

Departments in which supervisors fail to promote and provide opportunities for staff development and organizations that fail to support staff development are generally stagnant in other ways and may have difficulty recruiting and retaining high caliber staff (or sufficient staff if competition is keen). Recalling the earlier discussion on job satisfaction, the setting that fails to provide opportunities for staff development will, as a result, fail to provide the motivators that are important to job satisfaction and that may have much to do with retaining employees.

Some continuity in the work force of a department is essential. Too little is chaotic, and too much is deadening. Rapid turnover requires investing too much time too often in "breaking in" new employees who leave before they become fully productive. Little or no turnover closes off opportunities for advancement and may build up a resistance to change. Staff development cannot take place in the former environment and may wither in the latter environment.

Retention, turnover, and the implications for staff development can vary with the several levels of employee positions.

Employee Levels

As a general rule-of-thumb, employees in lower level positions tend to stay with an organization if their wages are competitive and if the work environment meets their social needs. These employees tend not to be mobile geographically or vocationally. They may transfer from department to department within an organization, often without prejudice and for reasons of better pay or working conditions (e.g., to get away from rotation on night shift). Their opportunities for promotion are usually quite limited. Advancement for merit, or for merit and seniority, may be by upgrading of position, e.g., from Aide to Senior Aide, or from Clerk to Clerk II, with an enlargement of responsibility and decision-making authority. Any investment in further developing these employees' knowledge and skills provides a direct return to the organization because of their tendency to stay.

Employees at mid-level positions, defined here as including nonsenior professional positions, semiprofessional positions, and technical positions, present different considerations. On the whole, these employees are more mobile than those in lower level positions. Some are mobile geographically or between institutions in the same geographical location, e.g., physical therapists in the first two or three years of their work experience. Some are mobile vocationally, switching fields with or without additional preparation and usually in pursuit of satisfying higher level psychological needs. Some physical therapists, probably some physical therapist assistants, and some secretaries (especially those who hold college degrees in other fields) fall into this category. Some of these employees, especially physical therapists, are upwardly mobile because their talents and ambitions coincide with the opportunities for advancement in the organization and in the field. This latter group of employees represents the best investment potential for staff development from the standpoint of the organization, the department, and the profession. Earlier comments about the importance of staff selection should be kept in mind here.

Because we do not yet have valid predictors to be used in staff selection, all employees in these mid-level positions become a major target population for staff development efforts. Recognize, however, that they also pose the greatest investment risk to the organization because of their mobility. Opportunities for advancement through promotion or upgrading of positions are crucial for these employees. Without these opportunities, they may see little reason to participate in staff development or they may soon depart for greener pastures.

Employees in senior professional positions and so-called middle management positions have already demonstrated their talents, ambitions, and stability in the field if not the organization. Continuing development is equally important to satisfying their higher level needs and poses the highest likelihood of enduring benefit to the organization and the profession.

Principles of Employee Development

Employee development has been defined as human growth which results from people coming into contact with new ideas (25). This development should be viewed not as a goal in itself, but as a means to an end. It should prepare the individual not only to perform all aspects of his present role, but, more importantly to be aware of the need to alter his style according to the changes that may be required at a later time. Growth for the future requires the development of conceptual skills, thereby providing for the necessary flexibility and adaptability. What is involved in the growth process is the challenge to convert methods-oriented youth into mature well rounded adults—adults who can proudly take their places in positions of responsibility in a rapidly changing world of health delivery. Development cannot be allowed to become a one-shot affair. It ought to be encouraged to continue throughout the individual's entire career.

That the capacities, abilities, experiences, and temperaments of no two people are alike is recognized by organizations. Hospital and agency-based programs are now concentrating on tailoring development programs according to individual needs of the departments and the people themselves.

When a supervisor hires an employee it must be remembered that he hires the whole person, with all of his strengths and all of his weaknesses. The greatest mistake that can be made is to attempt to build on known weaknesses. We should only build on known strengths. Appraisal then must aim more at bringing out what a person can do, rather than what he cannot do. This places a tremendous amount of responsibility upon the supervisor to take a more enlightened interest in the individual and to do a more competent job of appraisal, guidance, and development.

The planning of individual development programs must be performed by each supervisor working cooperatively with each subordinate. Results of previous performance appraisals will indicate strengths and weaknesses that should be used to guide the supervisor. To try to force every supervisor or potential supervisor into the same mold is unwise. We should not by our counseling or in our coaching attempt to remake our subordinates into our own image or try to force upon them a particular temperament or personality.

Supervisory training and staff development are intimately related to the entire system of practice in an organization. If administration is ignored, is disorganized, or is haphazard or faulty, staff development will be impossible to accomplish. Supervisors and staff learn to a great extent by example.

Hospital departments and other health care agencies must develop a policy toward organizational and employee growth. If this policy is a positive one, there is little doubt that an atmosphere of encouragement is engendered in the employees. This encouragement leads to a greater willingness to assume responsibilities and become ready by choice for advancement. Nothing is more frustrating than working in an organization or for a boss who disregards initiative and discourages growth. The supervisor helps create a climate for growth for subordinates in his relationships with them on a daily basis and can aid young people to realize their best potential. However, in the final analysis, the individual employee must want to grow. This can be demonstrated to the supervisor by undertaking a program of self-development. Such development occurs through participation in formal courses of instruction as well as on-the-job experiences. The role of the hospital or agency is to provide the atmosphere as well as the opportunity for its people to develop.

It must be clearly understood, however, that, regardless of the mechanism used, simply exposing staff to lectures, case studies, journal clubs, and job rotations does not guarantee that they will learn. The organization is important to this process, but equally involved is the worker himself, who must make the major effort in this regard. Self-development is the important concept in the whole program of staff and supervisory development.

Staff development and supervisory training must be undertaken on behalf of and by all members of the group, not by and for a chosen few. An organization will stand or fall on the basis of the total effort of the entire group. What must be developed is a multidimensional program that reaches to every supervisor and every staff member and helps educate in a variety of ways for a variety of specific purposes.

A program of staff development, to become effective, requires the support of the various levels of management in the organization. What must follow, of necessity, is an analysis of the needs now, and in the future, for the organization. Where will we be five years hence? What trends today may have impact on our needs for tomorrow? Once the data and the people are available, a concerted effort must be made to set up training programs and development opportunities.

Two principal concomitant ways exist by which people can acquire the knowledge, skills, and attitudes to become competent supervisors. One is through formal training and education courses; the other is through on-the-job experiences. Formal course work is an invaluable aid for learning new knowledge and new techniques and for broadening one's vision. Real learning, however, can occur only when the learner has an opportunity to practice and apply ideas. This learning can only be done on the job. If I were asked to specify which of the two influences carried the greater impact I would answer that on-the-job development is more important by far. One cannot place sole reliance on this particular method, however. Many supervisors are themselves not qualified to carry out this task. They may lack skill, interest, or the necessary patience. They also may possess erroneous notions of what administration encompasses. When on-the-job development is properly balanced with classroom learning, and when both are carried out in an atmosphere of sound management, a workable formula for development occurs.

This chapter is not an appropriate place to discuss the principles of teaching and learning. The managers and supervisors who devise instructional programs as part of their employee development opportunities should take these principles into account. Schein presents a useful summary and discussion of these principles as they relate to employees in organizations (24, pages 34–42).

MANAGERIAL TECHNIQUE FOR EMPLOYEE DEVELOPMENT

Job Rotation

The transfer of staff from job to job and from unit to unit on a coordinated planned basis is a popular means of employee development among larger hospital or agency departments. When a staff member takes on a new post in such a program, it is no mere orientation assignment. He or she is placed in a staff position where he will be back-stopped by more permanent personnel who give the employee and the unit a steadying influence, helping to keep things running smoothly if some difficulty should be encountered. Job assignments under a rotational scheme typically last anywhere from six to nine months. As a person gains experience over a period of time, he can never really acquire the broad perspective and diversified skills needed for promotion, unless he is deliberately placed in different types of learning situations. The department must take action to provide a variety of job experiences for those judged to have the potential for supervisory positions. Job rotation helps with this need. It also serves to break down unit provincialism. Supervisors who have served in other units can understand better the reasons why a particular function must be done in a particular way. Inter-unit cooperation is enhanced, as is a broader tolerance for other departments. Job rotation can also inject new ideas into each unit and help new concepts become infused and diffused throughout the department.

Coaching

Coaching is a procedure by which a supervisor teaches job knowledge and skills to a subordinate. The supervisor indicates what is to be done and may suggest methods by which it may be done and then follows up with an explanation and corrects any errors. The objective is not only to teach and guide the subordinate in the performance of immediate assignments but also to provide him with enough diversified work so that he can grow and advance.

All supervisors should foster the training and advancement of those who work for them. This can be done in several ways:

1. Give the authority that goes with responsibility; don't just tell the employee what must be done.
2. A job that is seen as a challenge will motivate people to do more than they are now doing.
3. What one accomplishes is what should be used as a criterion for advancement and for salary considerations.
4. Problems and mistakes should be converted into opportunities to direct talent and should be viewed as necessary for the growth process.
5. The subordinate-supervisor relationship should be one of trust and confidence.
6. The growth process should be tailored to fit the needs of the individual.

Although a great deal of emphasis has been placed upon coaching as a staff development tool, it cannot stand alone. Staff development is primarily a device for insuring that individuals grow within the boundaries set by their jobs and their organization units. Coaching works best when used in conjunction with periodic formal classroom instruction and other types of training.

Understudy

In the understudy situation a person is in training to assume, at some future time, the duties and responsibilities of the supervisor. To make the assignment, the names of therapists whose competence matches the needs of each supervisory job are submitted for consideration by the supervisors; the selection is made by the physical therapy director with the mutual consent of all supervisors; and one among the subordinates is selected in each unit to serve as an understudy to the supervisor.

The understudy is taught to grapple with the problems that confront the supervisor each day by handling such administrative matters as the supervisor may choose to delegate. He is given opportunity under guidance to try out his leadership style and to sit in on various unit meetings in place of the supervisor. This method is a sure, practical, and quick way of training the senior staff member for the job of supervisor. It emphasizes learning by doing and relieves the supervisor of a heavy work load. Understudy guarantees to the organization that it will not be at a serious disadvantage if the supervisor should have an extended furlough, vacation, or illness or suddenly terminate employment.

Stretch Objectives and Vertical Loading

Ross has advocated setting each employee's expected results just high enough to produce mild stress, a technique he calls setting "stretch objectives" (23). He believes that stretch objectives are important to self-development but cautions against setting such objectives too high, in which case they can produce a negative attitude and a drop in performance. The same author has advocated what he calls "vertical loading," an enlargement of job responsibility and decision-making authority to meet the individual's skills, abilities, and potential. The best way to enlarge the job of a subordinate, he claims, is to delegate some of the manager's or supervisor's own duties to the subordinate. He contrasts this vertical loading to "horizontal loading" which is merely increasing the volume of work expected of the subordinate.

I close the chapter on this note. The primary goal of personnel management is not to get more work out of subordinates but to help prepare them for taking over in effective and humane ways. Achieve the primary goal, and productivity will follow.

References

1. Argyris, C.: *Integrating the Individual and the Organization.* John Wiley, New York, 1964.
2. Barnes, M.R., and Crutchfield, C.A.: Job satisfaction-dissatisfaction—A comparison of private practitioners and organizational physical therapists. Phys. Ther., *57:* 35–41, 1977.
3. Berelson, B., and Steiner, G.A.: *Human Behavior—An Inventory of Scientific Findings.* Harcourt, Brace and World, New York, 1964.
4. Brennan, J.: *The Conscious Communicator—Making Communication Work in the Work Place.* Addison-Wesley Publishing Company, Reading, Pa., 1974.

5. Brown, J.D.: *The Human Nature of Organizations*. AMACOM, American Management Associations, New York, 1973.
6. Do you know how to listen? American Management Association, *32* (8): 111–116, 1980.
7. Feitelberg, S.B.: Basic considerations of a job description. J. Am. Phys. Ther. Assoc., *46:* 383–386, 1966.
8. Fritz, R.: Rate yourself as a manager. Association Management, *32* (8): 107–109, 1980.
9. Herzberg, F., Mausner, B., Peterson, R.O., and Capwell, D.F.: *Job Attitudes—Review of Research and Opinion*. Psychological Service of Pittsburgh, Pittsburgh, 1957.
10. Herzberg, F., Mausner, B., and Snyderman, B.B.: *The Motivation to Work*. John Wiley, New York, 1959.
11. Hickok, R.J.: Participative supervision in physical therapy. Phys. Ther., *49:* 731–734, 1969.
12. Hire people who can grow. Nation's Business, *9:* 36–37, 44–46, 1961.
13. Holmes, T.M.: Supportive personnel and supervisory relationships. Phys. Ther., *50:* 1165–1171, 1970.
14. Janis, I.L.: Psychological preparation for post-decisional crises. In T.W. Costello and S.S. Zalkind, eds., *Psychology in Administration—A Research Review*. Prentice-Hall, Englewood Cliffs, N.J., 1963.
15. Likert, R.: *The Human Organization*. McGraw-Hill, New York, 1967.
16. Lister, M.J.: Performance evaluation of the new staff member. J. Am. Phys. Ther. Assoc., *46:* 387–390, 1966.
17. Marcus, E.E.: The physical therapist in supervision. J. Am. Phys. Ther. Assoc., *46:* 391–394, 1966.
18. Maslow, A.H.: *Motivation and Personality*. Harper and Row, New York, 1970.
19. Mayo, E.: *The Social Problems of an Industrial Civilization*. Harvard University Graduate School of Business, Boston, 1945.
20. McClelland, D.C.: *The Achieving Society*. Van Nostrand, Princeton, N.J. 1961.
21. McDaniel, L.V.: The critical incident method in evaluation. J. Am. Phys. Ther. Assoc., *44:* 235–242, 1964.
22. McGregor, D.M.: *The Human Side of Enterprise*. McGraw-Hill, New York, 1960.
23. Ross, J.E.: *Managing Productivity*. Reston Publishing Company, Inc., Reston, Va. 1977.
24. Schein, E.H.: *Organizational Psychology*. Prentice-Hall, Englewood Cliffs, N.J., 1965.
25. Schneider, A.E.: The dilemma of management development. Personnel Administration, *13:* 12–15, 1964.
26. Steve, L.: Labor negotiations and the director of physical therapy. Phys. Ther., *53:* 623–627, 1973.
27. Vroom, V.H.: *Work and Motivation*. John Wiley, New York, 1964.
28. Wood, M.L.: Appraisal of professional performance—One aspect of physical therapy administration. J. Am. Phys. Ther. Assoc., *42:* 565–569, 1962.
29. Zimmerman, J.P.: An inventory of management skills. Phys. Ther., *49:* 84–86, 1969.
30. Zimmerman, J.P.: Employee problems and the counseling interview. Phys. Ther., *48:* 1420–1423, 1968.
31. Zimmerman, J.P.: Principles of organization for physical therapy. Part I. Phys. Ther., *52:* 876–878, 1972.
32. Zimmerman, J.P.: Principles of organization for physical therapy. Part II. Phys. Ther., *52:* 972–975, 1972.

chapter 2

POLICIES AND PROCEDURES

James Roodhouse

Policies and procedures are administrative tools used to carry out effective and efficient management. The extent of the policies and procedures required for a physical therapy service will be dictated by the purpose, size, and complexity of the service. No physical therapy service can disregard the need for policies and procedures. A physical therapy service that is a component of an institution or agency will abide by the appropriate institutional policies and procedures, but there are activities peculiar to a physical therapy service for which specific policies and procedures must be developed.

POLICIES

Policies set forth criteria for what is to be done and explain what activities will be carried out. Policies can be viewed as regulatory in nature, as they set forth the regulations within which daily operations take place. Although final approval of policies is the responsibility of the administrative head of the service or institution, it is advisable for the supervisor to obtain input from staff personnel when developing or revising policies. In many instances, the supervisor is not as aware and knowledgeable of the details of day-to-day activities as are the staff members who perform these activities. This approach also stimulates staff interest and encourages participative management. The end result is usually policies of better quality than if developed by the supervisor unilaterally. Also, staff will be more receptive to regulatory policies and more willing to abide by them if they have had input into their development. Policies should be written and categorically assembled into a policy manual for quick and easy reference. To avoid subjective and inconsistent interpretation, policies should not be established on an oral basis. Written policies should be specific, concise, and understandable to all affected employees.

All existing policies should be reviewed at regular intervals and revised if indicated. This review should be done on a regularly scheduled basis, not on a haphazard basis. Periodic review of policies is necessary and required in a

39

health care provision system in which federal and state legislative mandates and accreditation standards place ever increasing requirements on the management functions of health services providers. To abide by these legislative mandates and accreditation standards, it is imperative that policies that guide management functions be kept current and applicable by continually updating them. Policies initiated voluntarily to facilitate good management functions should be reviewed regularly along with those needed to meet the minimal requirements of external third parties.

A physical therapy service should have a written statement of purpose that specifies the activities to be performed by the service. Policies related to these activities are necessary for sound administrative management. For example, if the statement of purpose says the physical therapy service will conduct clinical research, a written policy should exist for research.

There is no specific guide for development of policies that will apply universally to all physical therapy services. Each physical therapy service will have to evaluate its total operation and determine the policies that will be required to meet all components of its operation. The more common policies required by physical therapy services are listed and explained in this section. This list is not all inclusive, nor will all the policies be applicable to all physical therapy services.

Personnel Policies

Recruitment and Interview

A physical therapy service should have a policy setting forth the responsibilities and methods for recruitment of personnel. The policy should be specific in explaining such areas as reimbursement for interview expense and final decision for hiring. During the interviewing process, policies affecting employment should be explained in detail to the prospective employee. The policies of the institution and the physical therapy service that directly affect or relate to job performance should be explained to the applicant during the interview. The applicant should have no doubt about the regulatory policies he will be expected to perform within and abide by. The recruitment policy should include all requirements necessary for the service or institution to satisfy the employment regulations set forth by such legislation as the Equal Employment Act and the Age Discrimination in Employment Act. A supervisor should be completely familiar with the laws regulating recruitment and employment. The purpose of an interview is to afford an opportunity for the employer and potential employee to come together and to communicate and evaluate the potential benefits each has to offer. Because employment decisions are many times made on initial observations and judgments, the interviewing process is of utmost importance to both parties. A sound policy that determines who will do interviews and how they will be conducted can often determine the success or failure of the interview.

Pre-employment Physical Examination

A policy that each new employee have a physical examination is highly desirable. If the physical examination cannot be given before the employee starts work, it should be given as soon as possible after the start of employment and the employee should be informed in writing that continued employment is dependent on satisfactorily meeting the physical requirements for the job. The pre-employment physical examination affords protection for the employer and for patients, if the employee will have patient contact. Pre-employment physical examinations are invaluable in preventing workmen's compensation claims for physical problems that existed before employment started.

Orientation

A policy for orientation of each new employee is vital for good employee performance. The policy should make clear who is responsible for completing the orientation and when the orientation will be done. Complete orientation to all aspects of the new employee's working environment and conditions will help dispel the fear and apprehension associated with new employment. The orientation should include but not be limited to information on days and hours of work, dress code, location of rest rooms, meal facilities, pay days, sick leave, vacation, insurance and retirement programs, absence from work, health services, fire and safety plans, and requisition of supplies. The new employee should be personally introduced to all co-workers. A written copy of the personnel policies, fire and evacuation plans, operations manual, and any other pertinent information should be given to each new employee on the first day of work. Within a reasonable period of time the new employee should be required to sign a statement that he has received, read, and understands all the policies and procedures that were furnished on the first day of employment. This statement can be very useful if later disciplinary action is required or if an unemployment insurance benefit claim must be contested.

Probationary Period

Many employers have a predetermined probationary period policy for new employees. The probationary period is a trial and adjustment period for both the employee and the employer. Usually during this period either the employer or the employee can terminate employment without notice. The employee is not considered a permanent employee during the probationary period. The employer may withhold certain benefits, such as sick leave accumulation and insurance benefits, during this period. The probationary period can be for any established period of time, but as a rule it should not be less than one month or longer than three months. The employee's supervisor should make a performance evaluation at the conclusion of the probationary period and the evaluation should be discussed with the employee. At the conclusion of the probationary period, employment can be terminated if performance is unsatisfactory, the probationary period can be extended if conditions warrant, or the employee can be changed to a permanent employee status.

Transfers and Promotions

A policy explaining transfers and promotions within the physical therapy service should be available. This policy prevents misunderstandings by explaining how employees can apply or will be considered for transfers or promotions. The policy sets forth the conditions for transfer or promotion to a new position. For example, the employee may be required to serve a probationary period in the new position with an evaluation after the probationary period before the transfer or promotion is considered permanent. If a probationary period is required, the length of the period should be established before the responsibilities of the new position are assumed.

Performance Evaluation

Performance evaluations of employees are vital for optimum personnel management and professional growth. The performance-evaluation policy should be specific as to when the evaluations will be done, by whom the evaluations will be done, and how the evaluations will be processed and used after they are completed. Performance evaluations should not be done solely as a means to justify giving or not giving salary increases. A regular performance evaluation affords the employee and the supervisor an opportunity to communicate and discuss work performance and personal characteristics. The evaluation should also afford the employee being evaluated the opportunity to communicate feelings about the job and to make suggestions and recommendations. At the time of the performance evaluation, objectives to be accomplished within a certain time interval can be established and agreed upon. A standard objective evaluation form should be used. Areas to be covered in the evaluation should include all those pertaining to work performance and personal characteristics; for example, quantity of work, quality of work, cooperation, dependability, initiative, and job knowledge. Other areas to be considered in evaluating personal characteristics are absenteeism, personal appearance, rapport with co-workers, and attitude. The evaluation form must have a standard grading system that is used for all performance evaluations to ensure uniformity of the grading process. Although it is impossible to eliminate human judgment in the grading process, the grading system should be as objective as possible. The policy for personnel performance evaluations should include a requirement that each evaluation form be signed by the supervisor making the evaluation and by the employee being evaluated.

Salary

The monetary compensation that employees receive for job performance is of utmost importance to most employees. A salary policy that explains when and under what conditions employees will be considered for salary increases contributes to employee morale and job satisfaction, and it alleviates many of the problems otherwise encountered because of lack of information. A salary policy is not the same as a salary scale or range. Salary ranges may be changed without necessarily changing the salary policy that sets forth the conditions for receiving salary increases. To enable employees to know when they will be considered for regular salary increases, the salary policy should specifically state the time intervals, such as the end of the probationary period, semiannually, or annually. The policy should also be specific if conditions other than time intervals must be met. If employees can earn merit increases for exceptional performance, in addition to regular salary increases, the policy should specifically set forth the conditions for merit increases.

Hours of Work

Hours of work for all employees should be firmly established. If employees are required to work beyond their normal workday or workweek, this should be included in the hours-of-work policy. For example, if a physical therapist or physical therapist assistant is expected to work on Saturdays in addition to the normal workweek of Monday through Friday, this requirement should be included in the policy, along with the amount and kind of compensation that will be given for additional work. The policy should be specific as to which activities after normal working hours are compensable and which are not. As health professionals, physical therapists cannot always conform to specific hours or shifts of work. If personnel are expected to participate in after-hour activities such as staff meetings and in-service education programs, the hours-of-work policy must be explicit as to what personnel can expect in compensation and what activities they are expected to perform or participate in voluntarily.

Health Services

A policy on health services for employees should include the health services required for employment and the health services that will be provided by the employer. Required health services may include an annual chest roentgenogram, periodic physical examinations, and certain inoculations. The health policy should specifically state when the requirements must be met, who will pay for them, and what action will be taken if they are not met. The health policy should also specify the nonrequired personal health services that will and will not be provided by the employer.

Dress Code

A dress policy or code for all employees establishes the wearing apparel and personal grooming requirements of employees during working hours. If employees are required to wear uniforms, the policy should clearly state the type, styles, and colors permitted. These requirements should be established and explained for all levels of employees if their dress requirements differ in type and color. The dress policy should be just as specific for employees not required to wear prescribed uniforms. The style and, if indicated, the color restrictions should be stated. If there are restrictions or requirements for dress accessories such as jewelry, shoulder patches, or name badges, these should be included in the policy. Personal grooming requirements or restrictions should be explicitly stated. Some requirements will conform to usually accepted standards such as adequate personal hygiene, good repair of apparel, polished shoes, and well-groomed hair, but they nevertheless must be included in the dress policy. If there are specific restrictions, they must be included in the policy. A dress policy must be frequently reviewed because fashion changes will require revision. It is advisable for management to include employee representatives in formulating the dress policy.

Vacation

A vacation policy establishes the amount of vacation accrual for employees and conditions under which vacation time may be taken. If employees in different job classifications accrue different amounts of vacation time, this differential must be firmly established in the policy. The vacation policy should also establish the rate of accrual—that is, the periodic intervals during employment for which vacation credit is given—and the maximum accrual permitted. The policy should be explicit regarding the conditions for taking accrued vacation. If employees are permitted to take portions of their accrued vacation at different times, this should be explained. Conversely, if employees are required to take their accrued vacation at one time or if they are allowed to take vacations only at predesignated times, these restrictions should be spelled out in the vacation policy.

Sick Leave

A sick leave policy sets forth the amount of time an employee can be absent from work because of illness and still receive normal pay and the conditions that must be met to receive paid sick leave. The amount of sick leave credit given each employee and when it is given should be stated in the policy. For obvious reasons, sick leave credit is usually not given until after completion of the probationary period and credits are given at specified intervals thereafter. The sick leave policy should also specify the conditions that must be met to qualify for paid sick leave. Such conditions can include notification by a certain time (such as one-half hour before the start of the working day) that the employee will not report for work, physician's approval to return to work after certain illnesses, etc. The policy should also state whether unused sick leave can be accumulated. A sick leave policy should be specific and leave nothing to arbitrary judgment. The more explicit a sick leave policy, the less it can be abused. When developing sick leave and leave of absence policies, supervisors must be aware of the requirements of the Pregnancy Discrimination Act as set forth in P.L. 95-555 amending Title VII of the Civil Rights Act of 1964.

Authorized Leave of Absence

A policy regarding authorized leave of absence is essential for a physical therapy service. This policy covers all authorized leaves of absence not covered in the sick leave or vacation policies. An authorized leave of absence may be with or without pay and the policy should be explicit in explaining each situation. Circumstances that should be considered for this policy are educational and professional meetings, jury duty, military duty, extension of absence because of illness beyond accumulated sick leave, personal business, emergencies, deaths, etc.

Discipline

A departmental policy for disciplinary action is advisable. This policy should specify who will be responsible for administering corrective or disciplinary measures to each level or category of employees. The policy should not carry a negative connotation; rather, it should be an instrument to facilitate good management. Such a policy enforces the "one boss" concept and provides an administrative tool to control intradepartmental conflicts. If an effective discipline policy is established, there should be no doubt on the part of employees as to what action will be taken if violations occur. An example of such action is an oral discussion of a first violation, written reprimands for the second and third violations, and possible dismissal after two written reprimands for the same violation. If possible, the policy should include a statement that each written reprimand be signed by the employee and dated when the reprimand is discussed with the employee. The signed written reprimand is invaluable if an employee is dismissed and later files an unemployment compensation claim that the employer wants to contest.

Temporary or Part-Time Employment

A policy explaining the working conditions for temporary and part-time employees is essential. The salaries and benefits offered temporary and part-time employees are often different from those given permanent full-time employees or they may be a proration of the full-time salaries and benefits. The policy should clearly state what benefits will be given part-time and temporary employees.

Retirement

A retirement policy establishes the age limit at which employment must be terminated. Federal legislation in recent years has significantly restricted the flexibility of employers in establishing these age limits independently. The 1978 amendment to the Age Discrimination in Employment Act of 1967 raised the permissable mandatory retirement age to 70, effective January 1, 1979. Supervisors must be knowledgeable of all laws affecting retirement age and develop policies accordingly.

Termination of Employment

A termination of employment policy explains the conditions for terminating employment by both the employee and the employer. The policy establishes the requirements of employees who terminate employment, and whether they are to receive terminal benefits such as accrued vacation, insurance, and retirement program options, etc. The most common requirement is a specified advance notice of intention to terminate employment, and the specified time may vary with the level of the employee's position. An employee in a supervisory position may be required to give a longer notice than a clerical or supportive employee. The policy should also state the conditions regulating the employer's dismissal of the employee. These conditions should specify the reasons for termination and the rights of the affected employee, such as the right to appeal and rights to accumulated benefits.

Exit Interview

A policy requiring supervisors to conduct exit interviews with terminating employees can be a great benefit to the supervisor of the physical therapy service. Unless a fixed policy exists, an exit interview is seldom done. The exit interview should obtain information as to why the employee is leaving employment and, if possible, what the employee plans to do after termination. If employees are leaving because of salary, benefits, or working conditions, it is essential that this be known so corrective action can be taken if indicated. Employees are usually more vocal and forthright in their statements at termination than during employment. In some instances, it is more beneficial for someone other than the employee's immediate supervisor to conduct the exit interview. It is also advisable for the terminating employee's immediate supervisor to complete a terminal evaluation form at the time of termination. The standard evaluation form previously discussed can be used. This evaluation form should be made a part of the employee's permanent personnel record and is invaluable if the employee reapplies for employment in the future or if reference requests are received from potential employers. The exit interview policy should include a requirement that all terminating employees sign a statement as to why they are terminating employment. A standard form should exist for this procedure and, unless the employee is being dismissed by the employer, the form should include a statement that the employee is leaving voluntarily with the understanding that he can continue employment in his position if he wished. This signed statement is valuable if the terminating employee later files an unemployment compensation claim which the employer wishes to contest.

Expense Reimbursement

An expense reimbursement policy establishes the regulations for reimbursement of certain expenses such as travel, room, meals, and tips incurred in attending meetings. This policy can also state whether moving expenses are paid for new employees and the limitation, if any. The policy should state not only what expenses are covered as reimbursable but the limitation of amounts if limits are imposed.

Speaking Engagements

Employees of a physical therapy service are often requested to speak to lay and professional groups. Often the speaker is considered a representative of his employing institution, and, as such, his statements and comments are attributable to the philosophy and objectives of the institution. In some instances, it is advisable to have an established policy for speaking engagements that sets forth certain conditions and requirements such as approval of the text of a speech before it is presented. The policy should also cover related matters such as the reimbursement of expenses incurred and the retention of honoraria received.

Additional Employment

If there are restrictions regulating the employment or practice of personnel outside of employment with the physical therapy service, a policy designating such restrictions should be in effect. An employer cannot regulate the off-duty activities of personnel; however, the employer can reserve the right to prohibit additional employment or practice as a condition of employment if desired. A policy is needed only if the employer elects to prohibit such outside employment or practice. If a policy is indicated, it should specify the type of employment or practice that is prohibited. Such restrictions are usually limited to kinds of employment or practice that pose a conflict of interest with the employee's regular employment.

Referral Policy

A physical therapy service should have a written policy clearly stating the conditions required for referring patients for evaluation and treatment. The policy should clearly state the sources from which referrals will be accepted, the method of referral required, and the information required in the referral. In developing the referral policy, the physical therapy service director must be cognizant of professional association ethical requirements and restrictions imposed by state and federal laws and regulations. The referral policy for the physical therapy service should be distributed to all potential referral sources.

Discount Policy

If the physical therapy service provides services at a discounted rate to certain individuals or agencies, a discount policy is essential. A physical therapy service that is a component service of an institution or agency will abide by the institutional or agency discount policy. A discount policy should list by category the persons or agencies entitled to discounted rates and the amount or percentage of discount allowed for each. Discount policies can carry certain stipulations. For example, a discount policy can carry a stipulation that, if a patient eligible for a discount has health insurance, the discount will apply only to the amount of charges not paid by insurance. The discount policy should be equitably applied to all eligible patients and strictly adhered to.

Affirmative Action

Physical therapy services that individually, or as a component service of a larger institution or agency, must comply with Executive Order 11246 must have and abide by an affirmative action plan. The supervisor of a physical therapy service that must comply with this order should be knowledgeable of its requirements. This policy must clearly state the personnel recruitment and employment practices put into effect to prohibit discrimination. The policy must be results-oriented and the policy should indicate who is responsible for the plan's implementation and fulfillment. The affirmative action plan must be publicized and distributed to sources from which referrals for employment will be received. Additional information regarding requirements for an affirmative action plan can be obtained from the Department of Labor.

Equipment Maintenance

An established policy for equipment maintenance is essential for a physical therapy service. This policy is required by accreditation and licensing bodies. A maintenance policy provides assurance that equipment is properly calibrated and meets optimum operational standards. This policy should specify that new equipment is checked and calibrated, if necessary, before being used for patient treatment. The policy should also specify the preventive maintenance program that will be done, who will do it, and at what intervals. Records of the maintenance program must be retained for accreditation and liability purposes. The maintenance policy should also specify the equipment to be cleaned on a routine basis and the checks to be made to assure effective results such as a periodic microbe culture of hydrotherapy equipment. State and local health laws that affect the physical therapy service should be reviewed and requirements that pertain to operation of the physical therapy service must be included in the policy.

Medical Records

A policy for medical records establishes what the records will contain and who is routinely privileged access to the records. The policy also explains the requirements that must be met before information is given to those not privileged routine access and the method of record retention. Laws and regulations will dictate to some extent what this policy will contain. Standards and accreditation commissions will also require certain conditions to be met. The physical therapy director should be knowledgeable of all conditions that affect record compilation and control. For example, the laws of some states provide that certain third parties may have access to a patient's record without the written authorization of the patient. The supervisor must know and be aware of all these conditions. The supervisor of a service that provides in-patient and out-patient services may be concerned with two records: the institutional medical record and the department record. The medical records policy should specify the requirements for record retention including the duration of time and the method of retention such as original record, microfilm, etc.

Summary

Policies are an essential management tool, and no service can effectively and efficiently operate without them. Accreditation commissions and regulatory bodies regard policies with such importance that they mandate their existence to meet standards and regulations or codes. To be an effective manager, a supervisor needs to know explicitly what is to be done and when it is to be done. Written policies that are current, applicable, and effective will provide this management tool. Basic policies that should be considered for effective management of a physical therapy service have been briefly explained. These policies are not intended to be all inclusive, nor are they intended to be applicable to all physical therapy services. The physical therapy service that is a component of a larger institution or agency need not be concerned with all policies, as many of them will be developed on an institutional or agency basis and will be applicable to the physical therapy service. It must be re-emphasized that to be effective, policies must be written and distributed to all indicated personnel. Operational policies cannot be oral agreements subject to individual interpretation. Such policies are as ineffective as no policy at all. Once written policies are in effect, they must be periodically reviewed, revised, and updated as indicated. The physical therapy service director must establish specific times when this review is to be done. Obsolete policies are not only inapplicable, they also reflect inefficiency on the part of the supervisor. As services grow and expand, as new employee benefits are given, and as new regulatory legislation is made effective, policies must be reviewed and revised as indicated. The important element is that the director of the physical therapy service should carefully and regularly analyze the operation of the service, review the policies that are in effect, and identify the areas that need policy development or change.

PROCEDURES

As policies set forth what is to be done, so procedures set forth how things are to be done. A procedure is a particular course of action or way of doing something. Because a procedure explains the details of exactly how something is to be done, it is usually more detailed than a policy and may even be a detailed elaboration of the policy itself. Although a corresponding policy is not necessary for each procedure developed for the physical therapy service, a procedure should be developed for each regulating policy if the policy requires certain activities for its fulfillment. Organizing written procedures into a procedure manual will enable all personnel to have an understanding of the total operation of the service and to relate their duties and responsibilities to that operation.

In developing procedures, the service supervisor should develop a standard format and use this format for all procedures. The procedure should be clearly identified by title. The text of the procedure should state precisely how the activity is to be done and the order in which it is to be done if several steps are involved.

Every physical therapy service should have written procedures to cover the basic application of certain treatment activities that vary little if at all. The physical therapy service supervisor should analyze all treatment activities and determine those for which written procedures are needed. Written procedures should not be regarded as a restriction of the professional judgment of staff but as a method of maintaining uniform application. There are records of liability claims being filed by injured patients because written treatment procedures were not available to personnel working in the physical therapy department. Some of the treatment activities for which written procedures should be considered are heat application, possibly massage, transfer of patients, and traction. If some of the treatment activities are performed by supportive personnel, written procedures are necessary to maintain uniform application and to aid in the training programs for these workers. The primary concern of the service supervisor should be patient safety and quality assurance. The development of written procedures specific to certain treatment activities may eliminate many of the variables that contribute to unsafe practices and inferior quality. It is certainly not indicated or necessary that written procedures be established for all treatments performed by professional personnel.

In addition to written procedures for certain treatment activities, the supervisor of the physical therapy service must have written administrative procedures if he is to maintain control of the management functions. These procedures indicate how administrative functions will be performed within the service.

As previously mentioned, each supervisor must analyze the functions and activities of his service and develop written administrative procedures as indicated. Some basic administrative procedures common to physical therapy services will be explained. These procedures are not intended to be all inclusive, nor are they intended to meet the requirements of every physical therapy service. Physical therapy services vary in purpose, composition, size, specialization, and structure, and the need for administrative procedures will vary accordingly.

Personnel

Many procedures are needed to implement personnel policies. These procedures can be so many and so varied, with large numbers of them already set down by institutions, that no attempt is made in this chapter to identify and explain them. A physical therapy director will have to analyze the service's operation and identify those personnel areas requiring procedures. A good method to follow is to identify all existing personnel policies (see, for example, the personnel policies discussed earlier in this chapter) and determine which ones need corresponding procedures for their implementation. Some examples are procedures for submitting and processing vacation requests, requests for attendance at educational conferences, and requests for approval of speaking engagements.

Referral

A physical therapy service needs an established procedure indicating how patient referrals will be processed. The policy on referrals will indicate the conditions for acceptance of a referral, and the referral procedure will describe how a referral will be processed after it is received. The detail of this written procedure will depend directly on the organizational structure and complexity of the service. If the physical therapy service is a component of a multiservice rehabilitation unit, there may be a central receiving department for referrals; the physical therapy service may not be too involved in the first steps of the procedure. Even so, the procedure must be understood and followed by physical therapy personnel to enable them to initiate it when referrals are received directly by them. If the referral policy states that oral or telephone referrals are accepted but that the referral must be countersigned by the referring physician within a specified period of time, the written procedure must include the ways and means of getting this accomplished. A referral procedure should include all steps of processing from the time the referral is received.

Records

Because a chapter on records is presented elsewhere in this book, the need for and use of records will not be discussed here except to state that a written procedure for compilation, control, and storage of records is advisable. The amount of information to be placed in the patient's record is determined by the service or institution. A procedure should be established specifying where and in what order this information will be placed in the record. To provide the supervisor with administrative control, the written procedure should include the personnel responsible for the various record activities.

Statistics

A physical therapy service should compile data and summary statistics regarding patient services. The data can be compiled on an activity form which can be consolidated into monthly and annual summary reports. Data to be considered are those on kinds and numbers of diagnoses, numbers of treatments given by modality, patient results, numbers of in-patients and out-patients served, etc. Summary statistics in the form of monthly and annual totals and averages provide a department director with information needed for effective management and planning. These statistics will be valuable in planning for department needs in such areas as personnel, equipment, physical facilities, and new service programs. The written procedure should explain what data will be kept, how they will be recorded, and summarized, and who is responsible for obtaining, recording, and summarizing the information. With ever increasing requirements being placed on treatment goals and results by third party payors, the availability of this information is of extreme importance. These data and statistics are also valuable for performing audits or for ongoing program evaluation.

Fire and Evacuation

A fire and evacuation procedure is a detailed statement explaining exactly what is to be done by each worker in the service. There are usually two procedures, one for fire and one for evacuation, although they may be combined in the same document. A fire does not always require evacuation, so workers must know what to do in case of fire alone and what to do if evacuation of the facility is indicated. A fire procedure or plan should indicate exactly what is to be done when a fire is discovered. This will be determined by the fire control system of the facility. The procedure may be calling a certain location for sounding a general alarm, tripping a fire alarm box, or possibly calling the fire department directly. Whatever method is used by the facility, it must be written, and every worker must know exactly what to do. The procedure must also state how to make a general alarm which notifies all workers that there is a fire and where it is located. One of the best methods for doing this is over a public address system. If there is no public address system, an alternative method of notification must be chosen. In small departments, a vocal announcement that will be heard by all may be sufficient. In larger departments some type of system has to be developed. If the service supervisor has any questions about developing a fire procedure, he should contact the local or state fire marshal who will be most willing to assist in development of the plan. When developing the plan, it is advisable not to use the word "fire" for sounding the general alarm so as not to promote panic and chaos. A phrase such as "red alert" or "emergency" is less excitable and conveys the message, and can be specified as the general alarm term in the fire plan. The fire plan should state what employees are to do when the alarm is sounded: this usually includes methods for putting out or confining the fire, removing patients from the vicinity of the fire, and reducing electrical hazards in areas of potential fire and water damage. The fire plan should state specifically where employees are to go and what they are to do in the event of a fire. The procedure may state that some employees stand by at specified stations for further instructions while others may be assigned specific duties such as obtaining a certain fire extinguisher and going to the location of the fire to help with a certain fire hose. The procedure has to be explicit and cover every detail so that each worker in the service performs without hesitation in this time of emergency.

The evacuation procedure or plan describes how all patients and workers will be evacuated from the premises if this becomes necessary. Evacuation can be the second phase of a fire plan if a fire reaches such magnitude that the safety of patients and employees is endangered. Evacuation may be required by an emergency other than fire, such as a bomb threat, and it may be necessary to put the evacuation plan into effect without a fire alert. Before an evacuation plan can be written, the supervisor of the physical therapy service must analyze the physical facilities of his department. He must determine where the exits leading outside the building are located. He must determine the closest outside exit for each room or area and who will use each exit to prevent traffic congestion during evacuation. After this has been determined, specific assignments of responsibility can be made. Each worker should be assigned to go to a certain area to assist in evacuating patients from that area and to leave the building after that area is evacuated. The evacuation plan should assign one person to check each area after everyone is evacuated, to ensure that certain things have been done such as shutting off all fans and blowers, turning on all lights, and closing, but not locking, fire doors. An out-patient physical therapy service should have current arrangements with nearby facilities for temporary shelter of patients and staff during an emergency requiring evacuation. Institutions should have arrangements for the temporary shelter and care, or transfer if necessary, of hospitalized patients if evacuation of facilities becomes necessary.

The fire and evacuation plans required will vary with each department and institution, but the important thing is that the plans exist and that they are current and effective. Practice drills for both the fire and evacuation plans should be held at frequent intervals to assure their effectiveness should an emergency occur; these drills should be integral elements of the plans.

Other Emergency Plans

Depending on local conditions or geographical location, a physical therapy director may need to develop plans and procedures for emergencies other than fire, for example, tornado, hurricane, flooding, and nuclear emergencies.

Disaster Plan

If a physical therapy service is a component part of a hospital that provides acute medical services, it will probably be included in a disaster plan. A disaster plan may be developed for an institution either independently or as part of a total community disaster plan. A disaster plan usually includes use of the physical therapy department physical facilities for predetermined services. The plan also includes the services to be provided by physical therapy department personnel in the event of a disaster. The physical therapy service supervisor must be knowledgeable of the disaster plan and how his facility and personnel will be used. All physical therapy service personnel must be aware of where to report and the duties they are to perform in the event of a disaster requiring their assistance.

Safety

Safety procedures must be established in a physical therapy service. Not only are these procedures indicated for employee and patient safety but many are required by the Occupational Safety and Health Act of 1970. The supervisor of the physical therapy service must be familiar with all requirements set forth in this Act, copies of which can be obtained from the United States Government Printing Office. Independent procedures need not be written for all safety considerations, but a safety element should be included in all appropriate treatment and administrative written procedures. For example, a written procedure for transferring patients can include statements on how to lift patients safely and on locking the wheels of wheelchairs when patients are transferred. The storage of flammable materials, grounding of electrical equipment, maintenance of nonslip floor surfaces, and security of wall-mounted and ceiling-mounted equipment deserve special attention in the safety procedures of the physical therapy service. The safety of patients and employees must be of primary concern to all employees of the physical therapy service, and the supervisor must provide the leadership and mechanism for its continued application. To assure compliance with the safety procedures, on-going safety programs and demonstrations can be carried out in the physical therapy service. If the physical therapy service is large enough, it is often advisable to have a safety committee, consisting of different levels of employees, that is charged with conducting and evaluating the safety program and procedures. The hospital safety engineer, local fire officials, and liability and workmen's compensation insurance carriers are usually very willing to work with the safety committee in developing evaluation and educational programs.

Accident and Medical Incident

A written accident and medical incident procedure states exactly what is to be done in the event that an accident or a medical incident happens to a patient or an employee. The first step in the procedure will usually depend on the availability of medical services. In a hospital setting, the person can be checked on site if physicians are present within the service, or the person can be taken to the emergency department. Whatever procedure is established, all employees must know what they are to do. If possible, all injuries should be checked regardless of how minor they are or appear to be. This precaution not only is advisable for the welfare of the patient or employee, but it also protects the treating employees and the service or institution if a liability suit is later filed for the injury. This precaution is certainly necessary for injured employees because of the reporting requirements of the Occupational Safety and Health Act (OSHA) of 1970. The supervisor of the physical therapy service must make certain the written procedure requires completion of an incident report within a specified period of time and states who is responsible for completing the report. For patient incidents or injuries, a copy of this report should be retained in the patient's medical record and other copies distributed as required. For employee incidents or injuries, a copy of the incident report should be retained in the employee's personnel or health file. The service supervisor must also be aware of other reports and the time restrictions for their preparation that may be required by OSHA, by the institution's insurance carrier, or by the state's employment or labor department or administration.

Financial Records

A physical therapy service that is a component of an institution or agency employing the service's personnel usually will not be concerned with financial records except for making daily treatment charges. If this is the service's only financial activity, a written procedure needs to be established explaining how treatment charges are made and how they are forwarded to the accounting or other indicated office.

Independent services and services under contract will be required to produce and maintain many varied financial records which will include treatment charges, periodic and annual financial statements of income and expenses, budgets, tax reports, reimbursable cost statements, audits, etc. The financial records required will in part be determined by the type of patient served by the physical therapy service. For example, if patients of a public assistance agency are treated, the service may be required to maintain certain financial records peculiar to that agency. There are certain requirements placed on providers of physical therapy services that provide treatment to Medicare patients. The supervisor of the physical therapy service should be intimately aware of these requirements and establish policies and procedures to assure their fulfillment. The topic of fiscal management, with illustrations of financial records, is presented in Chapter 7 of this book.

Purchasing

A physical therapy service should have a written procedure for purchasing equipment and noninventoried supplies used within the department. Such a procedure provides the supervisor with administrative control and promotes employee efficiency. If employees know the procedure for obtaining needed materials, they can initiate the purchasing process with an efficiency that prevents confusion and avoidable delays. The most common method for purchasing is using purchase requisitions and purchase orders. Any employee can initiate a purchase requisition which is forwarded to the supervisor of the physical therapy service. To maintain control of purchasing, the procedure should emphasize that all purchase requisitions must be written and must be approved by the service supervisor. If the physical therapy service does not issue the purchase order, the approved purchase requisition is forwarded to a central purchasing department that issues the purchase order. If the physical therapy service has responsibility for purchase, the written procedure should state who has authority to issue purchase orders and how they will be issued. If purchase orders are issued by the service, the procedure should also state how the vendors will be selected. For services having purchasing authority, it is advisable to maintain a petty cash fund for incidental and emergency purchases. The written procedure should also state how purchasing and reimbursement from the petty cash fund will be authorized.

Equipment and supplies are a major cost factor in the operation of a physical therapy service. Costs must be controlled and effective purchasing procedures are the manager's tool for controlling costs and obtaining the best prices available.

Supplies Requisition

A written procedure for requisition of inventoried supplies is required if the physical therapy service obtains expendable supplies or sells certain items of equipment that are not charged as an expense until requisitioned. The procedure for controlling requisition can be as lenient or as rigid as the supervisor desires. The preferred procedure is one of leniency so as not to deter or delay operation. The object of a requisition procedure is not to restrict but to control. A written procedure for requisitioning supplies provides employees with an organized method of obtaining materials necessary for day-to-day operation and yet provides the supervisor with the controls needed to fulfill supervisory responsibilities.

Equipment Maintenance

A written procedure for maintaining equipment in clean, sanitary, and working condition is a basic requirement for a physical therapy service. The procedure will include, for example, how equipment will be kept clean and sanitary. In this respect, the written procedure must state explicitly that equipment will be cleaned, how often it will be cleaned, and with what it will be cleaned. For example, the procedure can state that all hydrotherapy equipment will be drained and cleaned after every treatment with a certain specified solution or that paraffin in the paraffin bath will be changed at certain intervals. The equipment maintenance procedure is important and is effective for maintaining an efficient, sanitary, and attractive department. It is the responsibility of the physical therapy service supervisor to maintain the service in an effective and efficient manner which not only assures patients of quality service but also contributes to high employee morale. The supervisor must analyze the activities of the service and develop the equipment maintenance procedures necessary to accomplish this end result.

Summary—Procedures

Some of the basic procedures to be considered for a physical therapy service have been presented. Whether the procedures presented or others are indicated for a particular physical therapy service will have to be determined by the service supervisor. The supervisor must analyze every activity of the service's operation. As previously stated, policies must be developed first to establish what will be done. Then, development of procedures explaining how every activity will be done provides the supervisor with the basic management tools required for effective and efficient operation. By accepting the supervisory position, the supervisor accepts the management responsibilities for directing and controlling every aspect of the physical therapy service. Although the supervisor can delegate some of these responsibilities and the authority required for their fulfillment, the final responsibility remains with the supervisor. Procedures can be the most useful management tool a supervisor possesses, if they are developed wisely and used effectively.

After policies and procedures have been written and put into operation, they should be assembled into a manageable form. An effective method of accomplishing this is to develop an operations manual that includes, among other things, the policies and procedures that directly or indirectly affect all employees. The operations manual can also include other materials important to every employee, such as organizational charts and job descriptions. An effective operations manual will have four sections: (1) organizational charts, (2) job descriptions, (3) personnel policies and procedures, and (4) other policies and procedures. This compilation provides employees with access to all materials in one operations manual. The operations manual also provides the supervisor a convenient means of periodic review of all materials. A copy of the operations manual should be available to every employee of the physical therapy service.

Specialized procedures are often advisable for certain parts of the physical therapy service. For example, if physical therapy aides or orderlies are employed in the physical therapy service, it may be advisable to have a procedure manual for them in addition to the service's operations manual. This procedure manual would pertain only to the job activities of certain employees and could include a multitude of activities. Examples of procedures for physical therapy aides are how linen will be put on treatment tables, positioning of patients, standard water temperature for hydrotherapy, methods of cleaning equipment, and handling of linen. Examples of procedures for orderlies are how to lift and transfer patients, use wheelchairs and stretchers, and put on and take off braces. This type of procedure manual is indicated for nonprofessional personnel who have been trained on the job. If volunteers are used in the service, it is advisable to have a separate procedure manual to cover their activities. The special procedure manuals indicated for a physical therapy service will have to be determined by the supervisor.

QUALITY OF CARE

Quality care should be of highest priority to every member of a physical therapy service. "Quality care refers to care that has the characteristics of excellence. The assurance of quality implies a commitment beyond the measurement and evaluation of quality; it implies a commitment to take corrective action if care does not meet the criteria of the quality" (1). Policies and procedures certainly become involved in any attempt to measure and assure quality. Ever increasing emphasis and requirements are being placed upon the health care services delivery system to measure and assure quality. Accreditation commissions require program evaluation systems with minimum standards, regularly scheduled audits, peer review of the professional service component, and corrective action for identified areas of weakness. Purchasers of services and licensing bodies require similar activities. It is impossible to satisfactorily meet these requirements without effective, corresponding policies and procedures. Designing a quality evaluation and assurance system that will apply universally to all physical therapy services is probably impossible. Each system must be developed to establish and measure criteria for the individual service. What is going to be done requires policy commitment and implementation, and how it is going to be done requires explicit procedures. The physical therapy service director and staff must first commit themselves to evaluating and assuring the quality of care provided by the service, then establish a policy of what will be done, and finally develop procedures for implementing the policy.

SUMMARY

Policies and procedures have been defined and their importance in the administrative and management process explained. The need for a physical therapy supervisor to develop and implement policies and procedures will depend on the institutional affiliation of the service. Physical therapy services that are components of larger institutions will be governed by many of the institutional policies and will be required to comply with many of the institution's procedures. Although institutional policies and procedures exist, there are policies and procedures peculiar to a physical therapy service that should be developed and implemented. Whether or not policies and procedures exist, it is the responsibility of the service supervisor to determine what policies and procedures are required for effective administration and to take the action necessary for their development and implementation. Some policies and procedures that are common to physical therapy services have been identified and discussed. The number and type of policies and procedures will be dictated by the purpose, size, and complexity of the service. A commitment to evaluate and assure the quality of care provided by the service will require effective, corresponding policies and procedures tailored to the individual service.

Reference

1. American Hospital Association: Quality assurance program for medical care in the hospital. 1972.

chapter 3

DEPARTMENT PLANNING, DESIGN, AND CONSTRUCTION

Charles M. Magistro

PERSPECTIVES

This chapter is intended to provide the reader with an understanding of the considerations and requirements essential to the planning, design, and construction of a physical therapy department. The content deals primarily with planning and design of a department for the general hospital setting. Most of the factors considered will be applicable to other specialized treatment facilities offering physical therapy and rehabilitation services.

No attempt is made to present a model department for a hospital of a given size. Each and every physical therapy program is an entity to itself, and each department must reflect the individuality of that program and meet the objectives of the service. A properly designed and appointed department reflects the clinical services rendered and facilitates the delivery of quality care in an efficient and economical manner. Designing a model department to meet the needs of all 200-bed or 300-bed hospitals would be a meaningless exercise.

Planning and Innovation

The importance of physical therapists having some basic knowledge in the area of planning and designing physical therapy facilities and becoming actively involved in this process cannot be emphasized enough. Physical therapists have an unusual opportunity to make major contributions in the planning process. The extent to which they involve themselves in this process depends on their interest and knowledge but they can expect to be ably assisted by health planners, hospital administrators, and hospital architects. Regardless of how well qualified any of these people might be, they cannot effectively plan for and design a facility without input from the physical therapist. Even if architects have had previous experience in designing physical therapy departments, they will still require direction to cope with the variations in approaches to the delivery of physical therapy services. The

59

author's personal experience has been that these other professionals welcome the contributions and innovative ideas of the physical therapist.

The need to be innovative and to take advantage of modern concepts of design technology and construction should not be stifled. One can be highly imaginative and still retain those essential requirements apparent in any well designed department. To innovate means "to introduce something new." This does not in itself mean that the idea has never been thought of before, only that no one has implemented the concept. The ability to innovate requires confidence which is acquired only after thorough understanding and research of what is to be introduced. If you are satisfied that the innovations will improve upon existing methods and costs can be justified, all that is required is courage to implement your ideas and translate them into "progress."

The need to be innovative extends also to the area of design and construction of equipment which, for the purpose of this chapter, can affect many of the considerations in planning and designing a physical therapy department. Again from the author's own experience, most equipment manufacturers welcome suggestions that might improve their products and sales and at the same time improve the delivery of physical therapy service.

Growth and Expansion

In past years, hospital-based physical therapy programs were not always located in areas designed for that purpose, and many hospitals did not have physical therapy departments. The picture has changed dramatically. In 1978, 79.8 percent of the hospitals reporting to the American Hospital Association operated physical therapy departments (2). The proportion was even higher, 87.5 percent, if the data from hospitals of less than 50 beds are not considered. The first figure, 79.8 percent, is double the figure reported in 1955. This growth and expansion was the result of several factors, most of which stem from the fact that physical therapy has become an important, integral part of health care.

Hospital accreditation agencies and state licensing bodies emphasize physical therapy in facility standards, and at least one state requires that all new hospitals of 100 beds or more include a physical therapy service unit (5, 6, 12). The boom in hospital construction and expansion between 1955 and 1975, partially financed by the federal government through Hill-Burton funding, no doubt helped the growth and expansion of physical therapy services in hospitals.

Constraints

Hill-Burton funding is no longer available. Studies indicate that in most areas of the country a shortage of hospital beds no longer exists, and in many areas a surplus of beds and duplication of services have contributed to higher hospital costs. A report to Congress by the Comptroller General of the United

States points out many shortcomings in the manner in which health facilities are planned and constructed (16). The federal government's concern with these events led to the National Health Planning and Resources Development Act of 1974 and creation of a national network of local Health Systems Agencies (19). Congress created these agencies in an attempt to limit the rising cost of health care by eliminating unnecessary and duplicative equipment and services. The agencies review major hospital purchases and expansion projects in their respective areas.

No doubt the planning and design of physical therapy departments in hospitals will be influenced by the Health Systems Agencies. Their activities may result in some constraints on growth and expansion, but at the same time they may be valuable sources of data needed to justify growth and expansion.

EARLY CONSIDERATIONS

Planning is one of the more important yet difficult aspects of any construction project and must be started long before construction is begun. The aim of planning is to conceptualize a program before it exists and to envision the type of facility required to meet the program needs. No clear-cut formulas exist to make the planning process easier and more reliable but a number of factors will, if properly investigated, help minimize errors in designing the new department.

Some of the difficulties encountered in planning will be significantly reduced if an existing department is being expanded because some historical basis of performance and utilization exists. When planning for a totally new facility, less tangible evidence is available. In either case, the secret to comprehensive planning is to investigate as many factors as possible which might have pertinence to the program under consideration. Each factor standing alone may not seem to have great importance, but a composite of all factors, if carefully investigated, will provide a fairly accurate assessment of what might be anticipated. The emphasis in the factors discussed below will be on development of a new program but much of the discussion applies equally well to expansion of or changes in an existing program.

Type and Size of Hospital

This factor is easily determined, but is often misleading in terms of future program development. The type of hospital and the nature of services offered will usually have more significance than size. For example, if the facility is a specialty hospital for orthopaedic problems, the physical therapy department would differ markedly from that in a hospital of similar size with emphasis in another specialty area. Also, some general hospitals stress one type of service more than others. A general hospital in one area may service a large volume of out-patients, whereas a similarly sized hospital in another area may serve few if any.

The estimate was made at one time that no less than 10 percent of general hospital in-patients will require physical therapy services (4). This percentage, if accurate, would be an important piece of tangible evidence on which to forecast in-patient treatment visits. In actuality, however, the percentage of in-patients receiving physical therapy in general hospitals varies considerably from setting to setting. These variations seem directly attributable to availability of services, medical staff indoctrination to physical therapy, and, of course, the efficacy of the program. The use of a percentage ratio can be misleading when planning for anticipated in-patient services in a physical therapy department. One should plan for a greater number of in-patient visits in a hospital of 300 beds than in a 100-bed facility, but there is no absolute ratio to rely on.

When weighing the importance of the type and size of hospital, one should not overlook what is planned for the future in terms of expansion or shifts in areas of service. Long-range master planning is essential and can have considerable impact on the location of the proposed department in terms of possible future expansion. If the demands for physical therapy services continue to increase, most departments in operation today will encounter the need to expand, or to relocate in order to expand, in the next few years (14). The opportunities to do so, however, may be fewer if the constraints mentioned earlier persist. A location that permits expansion should be an early consideration in the planning process.

If a hospital is expanding its physical therapy department, a careful review of previous utilization patterns will provide an accurate forecasting tool.

Population Characteristics

The characteristics of the population served by or in the vicinity of the hospital should be considered early in the planning process. Here again no absolute yardstick exists for predicting utilization of the proposed program, but certain clues or trends may emerge from a careful study of location and population characteristics.

Will the facility be located in an industrialized area, or is it to be located in one of the more rapidly developing suburban communities? If located in a heavily industrialized area, one might anticipate a fair share of out-patient industrial cases. If located in the suburbs, one would expect a greater portion of in-patients, since most people would rather be hospitalized nearer their residence. What have been the trends in population shifts in the area to be served? Has the population increased or decreased and at what rate? What percentage of the population is over age 65? Persons in the 65 and over age group are known to demonstrate a higher use of medical services than those under 65, especially for chronic conditions that accompany increasing age. Younger people, on the other hand, are more likely to demonstrate acute injuries from automobile, motorcycle, and skiing accidents, and even from jogging. Is the area an economically stable one? Is the community subjected to seasonal shifts in population? These examples and questions serve to illustrate the kinds of characteristics of the population and location that should be examined early in the planning process.

Federal and state agencies and their publications, as well as the local Health Systems Agencies mentioned earlier (19), are useful sources of the demographic data that should be examined. In addition, workloads of hospitals of similar size, locations, and missions should be studied. A review of these types of data will provide an overview of the location, the numbers, and types of people who will potentially be served by the physical therapy department.

Existing Services

The fact that other physical therapy services exist within the general area may have considerable influence on the scope of the program being planned. This influence interestingly enough may either enhance or decrease the utilization of the developing program. For the past several years, much effort has gone into comprehensive facility planning. One must commend the purpose of this program. Comprehensive facility planning, however, often neglects to consider factors which are so essential to the consumers of health services, such as availability, accessibility, and quality. These factors ultimately affect the use of the services, including physical therapy.

One must be totally realistic in the assessment of existing services and the impact that duplication of services could have on utilization. If well established and accepted programs are already available and are meeting existing demands, a marked shift of patients to a new department is unlikely. If physicians in the area customarily treat out-patients in their offices, this pattern of practice is unlikely to change markedly as the result of a new service being available. If definite voids exist in the types of services offered in the area, and if these voids can be documented, fewer problems with competing facilities and services will be encountered.

A careful review of all facilities and agencies that provide similar services should be conducted early. Attempt to evaluate the effectiveness of existing programs and their level of activity in realistic terms. This aspect of planning is important because it provides many clues in terms of defining the proposed department and its services.

Referral Sources

The number, types, and referring characteristics of physicians who might use physical therapy services in the proposed department, as well as possible referring agencies in the area, are basic considerations to be investigated.

One should expect that a review of the physicians who might use the service would provide some reasonable expectation of referrals. This is not necessarily true. Certainly one should expect more physical therapy referrals from an orthopaedist than from an obstetrician. But will the orthopaedist refer more patients to the program than the general practitioner? The answer will depend upon the referral habits of both physicians, and their knowledge of what value physical therapy services might provide their respective patients. The physician who is well versed in all aspects of physical therapy services is the unusual physician. Questioning an uninformed physician on how he might use the services would not provide reliable information.

Changes in Delivery and Practice

For a variety of economic and social reasons, the delivery of health care services is undergoing intensive study and rapid change. Utilization review and the development of Professional Standards Review Organizations have had noticeable effects on curtailing unnecessary admissions to hospitals, excessive lengths of stay in hospital, and overutilization of hospital services. Increasing emphasis continues to be placed on ambulatory care and health maintenance. Different levels of health manpower have been created to extend or assist the services of practitioners. Concern is growing that the nation may soon face a surplus of health practitioners, and controversy rages over whether this is good or bad for the cost and accessibility of health care. And restrictions on advertising by practitioners have been set aside or markedly reduced. All of these changes and events will affect the delivery of health care services, including physical therapy, both within and outside the hospital.

The physical therapist responsible for planning a new department, or planning changes in an existing department, must become informed early about recent and potential changes in the delivery of health care services, in general, and the delivery of physical therapy services, in particular. Going back to an earlier comment about innovation, the planner may want to consider implementing changes in the delivery of care that anticipate the future.

The practice of physical therapy, over and above any changes in the delivery of services, is also undergoing rapid change. Some of this change is the result of new knowledge gained through research, some is the result of technological advances, and some is the result of new, or changing, or more intensive areas of interest. New methods, new equipment, special expertise, and even the conduct of clinical research in the new department will affect its planning and design. Again, the physical therapist responsible for planning the department must become informed early about recent and potential changes in practice through research, technological advances, and areas of interest. Opportunities for innovation here should certainly not be overlooked. The early stage of planning is an excellent time to consider, for example, the anticipated clinical research activities or special clinical activities of the new department.

Services and Activities

Early consideration of the factors discussed above—type and size of hospital, population characteristics, existing services, referral sources, and changes in delivery and practice—leads quite naturally to the next early consideration: the services and activities of the proposed program and department.

Some, certainly not all, of the pertinent questions to be answered here are: Will the department provide mostly short-term care for acute problems, long-term rehabilitive care for severe disabilities, or some combination of both? If the plan is to become involved in long-term care of more severely disabled patients, consideration should be given to the size and type of gymnasium planned, the need for a well equipped area to conduct activities of daily living, and proximity to the department of occupational therapy.

Will the department provide mostly in-patient care, out-patient care, or some combination of both? The answer will have much to do with planning space to accommodate either wheelchairs and wheeled stretchers, ambulatory waiting space, or both.

Will the department be used as a clinical affiliation center for students? If so, provision must be made for charting space, lockers, and private study or discussion. Will the department conduct or participate in clinical research? If so, then provision must be made for special equipment, isolation from the noise and traffic of the rest of the department, and data reduction facilities.

These questions are posed only to illustrate some of the early considerations that need to be given to the anticipated services and activities of the new or expanded physical therapy department. The questions do not exhaust all of the possibilities that will influence the ultimate planning and design of the department.

FIRST REQUIREMENTS

After having carefully studied and made decisions about the early considerations discussed above, the planner should establish certain first requirements to assure that the services and activities can be conducted under optimal conditions for the efficient and effective operation of the physical therapy department. These first requirements are discussed below.

Accessibility

The department must be conveniently located if it is to serve both in-patients and out-patients. Proximity to hospital elevators is highly desirable in order to transport in-patients to the department. If out-patient services are planned, a first floor location with nearby reserved parking is recommended. Many hospitals find advantages in clustering their service departments such as radiology, pathology, pharmacy, emergency room, and physical therapy.

In this way common waiting areas, receptionist offices, and rest room facilities can be shared. The primary consideration, however, should be the fact that patients who need access to the physical therapy department are physically handicapped to various degrees, whether temporarily or permanently. An excellent reference source on accessibility requirements for the physically handicapped is available and should be consulted (18).

Whenever possible the physical therapy department should be located on the main floor of the facility. The importance of this location to the effectiveness and efficiency of the total program should not be underestimated. The scope and use of the program can be enhanced tremendously if the department is located within a prominent area of the hospital. Locating the physical therapy department in some remote section of the hospital or in the basement will seriously impede the potential use of the service.

Sometimes, because of hospital design or the characteristics of the physical therapy program, small ancillary physical therapy units need to be established on nursing floors. These units need not be pretentious and can serve as a valuable adjunct to the function of the main department. Definite consideration should be given to such units if programs are being planned for specialty care of burn, orthopaedic, stroke, coronary, or respiratory problems. Often, the condition of patients or the nature of their treatment program mitigates against their being transported to the main department for treatment. Making provision for storage of certain essential equipment on the various nursing floors may also be desirable. These storage areas will increase the efficiency and effectiveness of bedside treatment programs.

Functional Areas

The general hospital physical therapy department needs areas for at least four separate functions. The minimum required functional areas are a hydrotherapy area, a gymnasium, a treatment cubicle area, and an area or areas for support and other nontreatment purposes such as administrative, staff, student activities, patient waiting, storage, and restrooms. The planner may consider additional functional areas as being essential but the four mentioned are absolutely required for serving the program needs in a general hospital.

The amount of space allocated for each type of functional area will depend upon a variety of considerations. Factors such as the types of patients to be treated, anticipated utilization, constraints imposed by costs, and architectural barriers are but a few of the considerations. The topic of space requirements is discussed in detail later in this chapter.

The possibility and nature of future expansion of the department should be considered at this stage of the planning process (15).

Staffing

The number and types of professional and support staff needed to operate the proposed department is a first requirement that needs to be determined.

Ratios of staff to patient visits or treatments are difficult to ascertain, however, and, if ascertained, may be misleading. Many variables must be taken into account when attempting to determine the size and mix of personnel required to operate the department. Presently, very little reliable data is available to assist the planner in estimating staffing requirements. Attempts have been made to gather information that would reflect staffing patterns for institutions of comparable purpose. Because of the unreliable definition of what constitutes a treatment, however, these comparisons are meaningless and have been abandoned (3, 7, 17).

Three things are fairly certain in considering staffing requirements. The number of personnel in a developing physical therapy department can be expected to increase beyond the original size; the clerical demands on the service will increase, as they will for all health care services; and, personnel costs will represent the major annual expense of the department. The design of the department, therefore, should be one that contributes maximally to staff productivity in order to maintain personnel costs at a reasonable level.

NARRATIVE AND SCHEMATIC PRESENTATION

Some of the more important early considerations and first requirements in planning a physical therapy department have been discussed. After studying these factors and making the necessary determinations, the planner should have a concept of how the department will function and what will be needed to carry out these functions. This information must be formalized into realistic and measurable terms and transmitted in writing to the architects involved in the design of the department.

Narrative Proposal

The narrative proposal outlines in rather specific detail the planned program and how it will function. Decisions must be made about types of patients, accessibility, functional areas, services and activities, staffing, and possible future expansion. These decisions, which are still reversible at this point in time, and descriptions of what will take place in the department are included in the narrative proposal and communicated to the architect.

A complete narrative proposal will enable the architect to prepare schematic drawings which are the first step in a series of progressive developmental drawings of a construction project.

Schematic Drawing

A schematic drawing is nothing more than a diagram or scheme, not drawn to scale, showing the relationship and traffic flow among the various functional areas and other major elements of the department. A schematic drawing of the physical therapy department is shown in Figure 3.1. Notice that the drawing shows very little detail and only the approximate, relative size of the various areas.

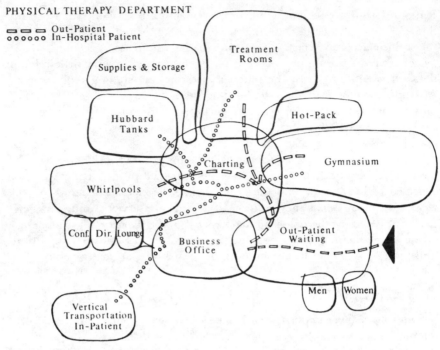

PHYSICAL THERAPY DEPARTMENT

▭ ▭ ▭ Out-Patient
ooooo In-Hospital Patient

Supplies & Storage

Treatment Rooms

Hubbard Tanks

Hot-Pack

Charting

Gymnasium

Whirlpools

Conf. Dir. Lounge

Business Office

Out-Patient Waiting

Men Women

Vertical Transportation In-Patient

Figure 3.1. Schematic drawing depicting the relationship and traffic flow among various department functional areas.

After studying the narrative proposal to learn how the department will function, the architect prepares the schematic drawing in order to arrange the various areas within the department so that traffic flow is orderly and cross-traffic patterns are kept to a minimum. These areas must be connected by means of a circulation system so arranged that when connections are completed, the department will function with maximum efficiency. A patient should be able to enter the department, register, go to the appropriate area or areas, be treated, check out, and exit in an orderly fashion.

SPACE REQUIREMENTS

Ultimately all effort expended in the planning process must provide information on the anticipated utilization of the service, one of the most important factors in determining space requirements. Regardless of how carefully one has studied all factors in the planning phase, total space requirements will to a certain extent represent some guess work. It is impossible to predict accurately the degree to which a new service will develop and be used. This section of the chapter offers some suggestions and considerations that will help reduce the guess work and improve the accuracy of space requirement estimates.

Defining Functional Areas

The four types of department functional areas identified earlier are presented in Table 3.1 along with the elements that define or make up the areas. Each element, with some exceptions (see footnote), is accompanied by suggested dimensions based upon the author's experience and drawings such as are shown in Figure 3.2.

The drawings in Figure 3.2 make clear that the dimensions of an element take into account the space required not only for equipment and furnishings but also for working efficiently around the equipment and furnishings.

Notice in Table 3.1 that the dimensions and square feet are given for only one treatment cubicle, an element in the Cubicle Area. For elements such as

TABLE 3.1
Functional Areas and Suggested Dimensions

Areas and Elements	Dimensions	Square Feet
	feet	*feet*
Cubicle Area		
Treatment cubicle	8 × 10	80
Examination/Special procedure room	10 × 10	100
Cubicle area work station		
Hydrotherapy Area		
Small whirlpool	5 × 7	35
Extremity whirlpool	7 × 8	56
Lowboy whirlpool	8 × 8	64
Hubbard tank	16 × 18	288
Hydrotherapy work station[a]		
Gymnasium[a]		
Administrative/Support Services		
Patient waiting[a]		
Reception/Business office	10 × 15	150
Director's office	10 × 12	120
Staff office	10 × 12	120
Staff lounge	12 × 15	180
Charting area[a]		
Conference Room/Library	12 × 15	180
Patient restroom	6 × 7	42
Staff restroom	5 × 6	30
Janitor closet	4 × 5	20
Staff lockers		
Storage[a]		
Clean linen		
Dirty linen		
Supplies		
Equipment		
Charts/Forms		
Wheelchair/Stretcher		

[a] See suggestions in text.

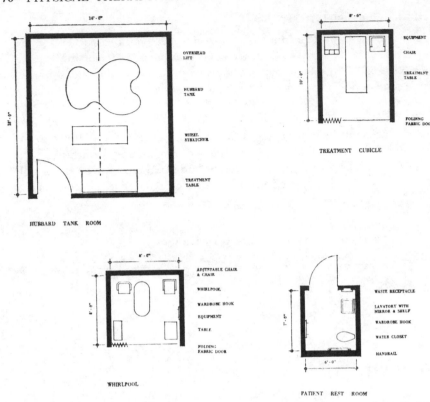

Figure 3.2. Dimensions of selected areas within a physical therapy department.

treatment cubicles and whirlpools, the obvious question about space requirements becomes this: How many will be needed?

Number of Functional Area Elements

The number of elements needed in a functional area, for example, the number of treatment cubicles needed, will depend upon the anticipated use of the particular element. Several methods for determining this need have been proposed (1, 10, 13, 14, 15), but these methods lack the comprehensiveness and accuracy of one proposed by Doctor (8). The method and worked example given below are based on Doctor's approach. The figures used are for illustrative purposes only. Actual figures could be obtained from data collected in a setting similar to the one being planned.

Assume first that the planning problem is one of determining the total amount of treatment cubicle space required, that is, the number of cubicles times space per cubicle. To estimate the number of cubicles needed:

1. Determine the average *occupancy time*, O, of a cubicle for treatment of one patient. Occupancy time, expressed in minutes, includes time required for preparation, undressing and dressing, and clean-up.

2. Estimate the total number of patient *treatments*, T, per day that will require cubicle space. A treatment is defined here as each occasion that a patient enters a cubicle, receives treatment in the cubicle, and then leaves.

3. Identify the total *available time*, A, per day that a cubicle could be used for patient treatment. Total available time, expressed in minutes, would not ordinarily include the lunch hour.

4. Determine the typical daily *utilization ratio*, U, of a cubicle. The utilization ratio is defined here as the proportion of daily available time (A) during which a cubicle is likely to be occupied (in use, being prepared, and being cleaned). This ratio is usually greater than 0.50 and less than 1.00 (treatment cubicle are rarely, if ever, in use during all of the available time).

Assume that the following figures have been obtained:

O (occupancy time)   =   30 minutes
A (available time)   = 420 minutes
T (treatments)   =   30 per day
U (utilization ratio) = 0.80

The number of cubicles or elements (E) needed is estimated by use of the formula:

$$E = \frac{TO}{UA}$$

For example, $E = \dfrac{30 \text{ treatments} \times 30 \text{ minutes}}{0.80 \times 420 \text{ minutes}} = 2.7 \text{ or } 3 \text{ cubicles.}$

If each treatment cubicle requires 80 square feet (see Table 3.1), then the total space required for treatment cubicles in the example is:

3 cubicles × 80 square feet = 240 square feet.

The method just presented is one way of estimating space requirements. That method relies on experience and data for figures to be inserted into the formula. Experience and data are valuable sources of information for estimating space requirements even when no formula is used.

The author studied numbers of daily patient visits, numbers of treatment

Table 3.2
Relationship of Patient Visits to Treatment Cubicles and Hydrotherapy Units (based on seven-hour day)

Number of Daily Patient Visits	Number of Treatment Cubicles	Number of Hydrotherapy Units
10–25	2–3	1
25–50	3–5	2 + Hubbard—Optimal
50–75	5–7	3 + Hubbard—Optimal
75–100	7–9	4 + Hubbard tank

Table 3.3
Space Planning Criteria for Full Time Physical Therapy Services (9)

Function	Basis for Planning	Space
		sq feet
Reception Area	1 per clinic minimum	110
Offices		
OIC	1 per clinic minimum	120
NCOIC	1 per clinic at 1200 visits per month	110
Staff Therapist	1 only projected	110
	2 or more projected	ea 85
Cubicle Area		
Cubicle	1 per each 400 visits per month.	120
	Minimum of two cubicles	
Cubicle Work Station	1 per each two cubicles	60
Exercise Area Stations	1 per each 200 visits per month.	60
	Minimum 6 stations	
	Maximum 18 stations	
Rehabilitation Area	At 350 visits per month (Parallel bars)	230
	At 800 visits per month (Parallel bars, mat and tilt table)	530
	At 1500 visits per month (Parallel bar, mat, tilt table, gait lane, exercise stairs and 20 SF gait training aids)	750
	At 2500 visits per month (above equipment plus a second tilt table, 30 SF)	880
	At 3500 visits per month (above equipment plus a second gait lane, 30 SF)	1000
Storage	10 per cent of the exercise and Rehabilitation areas. Minimum 60 SF	
Hydrotherapy Area		
Extremity Whirlpool	1 per each 500 visits per month	80
	Minimum 2 whirlpools	
	Maximum 7 whirlpools	
Lowboy Whirlpool	1 per each 800 visits per month	90
	Maximum 2 whirlpools	
Whirlpool Treament Cubicle	1 per each four whirlpools	120
Whirlpool Work Station	1 per each three whirlpools	60
	Minimum 1 work station	
Contour Body Tank	1 at 800 visits per month	235
	2 at 5000 visits per month	
Therapeutic Pool	At 1800 visits per month	2500

cubicles, and numbers of hydrotherapy units in a general hospital setting, based on a seven-hour working day. The results, presented in Table 3.2, may provide a quick and ready reference for some planners.

A highly detailed, comprehensive tabulation of space requirements, related

Table 3.3—*continued*

Function	Basis for Planning	Space
		sq feet
Waiting Area		
Spaces	1 space per each 200 visits per month	16 per space
	Minimum 5 spaces	
	Maximum 15 spaces	
Litter and Wheelchair Space	1 space per each 500 visits per month	25 per space
	Maximum 6 spaces	
Exam/Special Treatment Room	1 per clinic minimum	110
	2 at 2500 visits per month	
	3 at 5000 visits per month	
Wheelchair Restroom	1 per each clinic minimum	50
	2 at 1200 visits per month	
Dressing Booth	1 per each 800 visits per month	30
	Minimum 1 booth	
	Maximum 6 booths	
Patient Lockers	3 per each dressing booth	10
	Minimum 3 lockers	
	Maximum 18 lockers	
Staff Restroom	1 at 1600 visits per month	30
	2 at 3000 visits per month	
Staff Lockers	1 per each projected staff	10
Staff Lounge	A 800 visits per month	110
	At 1800 visits per month	120
	At 2500 visits per month	140
	At 3000 visits per month	160
	At 3500 visits per month	180
Clean Linen/Drying	1 per clinic minimum	80
Soiled Linen/Service Room	1 per clinic minimum	80
Janitor Closet	1 per clinic minimum	20
Special Treatment Programs		
Activities of Daily Living		150–300
Amputee Training		450–600
Cardio/Pulmonary		150–300
Electromyography		110
Pediatric Rehabilitation		150–300
Special Exam/Research		110–300
Clinical Education Program		
Education Supervisor Office		110
Conference Room and Library		200
Training Aids Alcove		50
Student Carrels	1 per each student	30

in large part to patient visits, was developed in the 1970s by a Tri-Service Physical Therapy Committee of the U.S. Armed Forces (9). The document, presented in Table 3.3, sets out space planning criteria for physical therapy departments in military installations but much of the content should be useful to civilian planners. Notice that the elements identified in Table 3.3 are organized for the most part according to types of functional areas, as in Table 3.1.

Occupancy Time and Space Requirements

For the formula and example given earlier, occupancy time was defined with specific reference to treatment cubicles. The definition, of course, can be extended to occupancy of any treatment, evaluation, research, or other special purpose space. Any extension of the definition should include preparation and clean-up time for a realistic estimate of space needs. For planning and other purposes, occupancy time can be subdivided to show attended and nonattended treatment time. A study done by Heath in three large naval hospitals shows the several components of occupancy time for an extensive list of physical therapy activities (11). The results of the study, presented in Table 3.4, provide sound estimates of occupancy time that can be used or adapted for a variety of settings.

Occupancy time should also be viewed from other prespectives if maximum use of planned space is to be achieved. The solution to meeting space needs does not always lie with acquiring more space.

Attempts should be made to alleviate congestion in treatment rooms. It is possible and sometimes advantageous to move patients out of selective treatment areas when a part of their treatment program has been completed. For example, the administration of sitting cervical traction or therapeutic exercises to a hand, or applying dressings, might just as easily be carried out in another area of the department freeing a treatment cubicle. These concepts must be anticipated and provisions made to carry them out.

Wall-mounted cervical traction units can be placed in recessed alcoves or in the gymnasium. Wall hung, collapsible hand exercise tables can also be located in the gymnasium. Dressing stations adjacent to hydrotherapy units will alleviate congestion of whirlpool areas.

The planner should also recognize that some patients will be treated at bedside only, and others will use only the gymnasium.

Available Time and Space

Available time, like occupancy time, was defined earlier with specific reference to treatment cubicles but can be extended to any space in the physical therapy department. Unlike occupancy time, however, available time depends upon the number of hours per day and the number of days per week that the planned department will be operational.

When considering space requirements for a new or expanding department, the planner should look carefully to the hours and days of operation as another alternative to acquiring more space. Space, equipment, and furnishings represent a costly investment. Once acquired, they "exist" 24 hours a day and seven days a week, or a total of 168 hours per week. Offering physical

Table 3.4
Time Factors for the Administration of Physical Therapy Services (11)

Attended Treatment Time The time required for constant attention with a patient by staff	Preparation and Clean-up Time This includes preparation of the treatment area and equipment, the application of equipment, removal of appliances and dressings, transportation of the patient, etc.	Nonattended Treatment Time This is the amount of time a patient spends receiving treatment exclusive of staff attendance and preparation and clean up time

All Time Values Expressed in Average Minutes

Description of Service	Attended Time	Preparation and Clean-up Time	Nonattended Treatment Time	Total Time
Evaluation and Treatment Planning	11	1	0	12
Electrodiagnostic Testing	34	7	0	41
Tests and Measurements	14	10	0	24
Home Instruction	16	5	0	21
Hot Packs	1	10	19	30
Infra-Red	1	10	19	30
Ultraviolet	20	15	0	35
Cryotherapy	13	10	0	23
Shortwave Diathermy	2	15	18	35
Microtherm	1	10	25	36
Ultrasound	11	10	0	21
Electrical Stimulation	12	10	0	22
Traction	2	5	20	27
Intermittent Compression	1	5	34	40
Arm Whirlpool	1	10	20	31
Leg Whirlpool	1	25	20	46
Lowboy Whirlpool	1	40	20	61
Hubbard Tank	25	45	0	65
Contrast Baths	1	15	24	40
Paraffin Bath	1	10	20	31
Comb. Ultrasound-Elec. Stim.	12	10	0	22
Therapeutic Exercises	8	10	0	18
Massage	12	5	0	17
Gait Training	17	10	0	27
Prosthetic Training	35	10	0	45
Self Conducted Exercise-Gait	4	1	20	25
Dressings	14	5	0	19

therapy services 35 or 40 hours a week, as is still common practice in many general hospital settings, means that this costly investment is available for use less than 25 percent of the maximum possible time.

Departments of the future, in order to maximize their utilization potential and reduce construction and operational costs, must give serious consideration to extending periods of service. For example, a department that normally operates on a seven-hour day (one-hour lunch break), five-day week schedule can increase its utilization by 30 percent by remaining open two additional hours and staggering the lunch hour. The available time would increase even more if out-patient services were provided on Saturdays and in-patients were treated on weekends.

Maximizing the use of space and equipment is not the only reason for extending periods of service. It is incongruous to think that a patient hospitalized for physical therapy should go without these services on weekends. Similarly, many out-patients find it difficult to leave their place of employment during normal working hours and would welcome extended hours or weekend services.

Today, departments are beginning to respond to these demands and are offering extended hours and days of service. Staffing requirements to meet these increased periods of service are being achieved through a variety of innovative staffing arrangements. These can include staggered hours of work, compensatory time off for staff work on weekends, the 10-hour work day concept, and use of part-time personnel.

The considerations about available time and space discussed above become even more important when one realizes that the space required for corridors, mechanical equipment, architectural obstructions, and accessways to the various functional areas will substantially reduce the overall useful space available to the department.

Finally, the concept of available space should not be confined to horizontal or floor space. The ceiling height in the Hubbard tank area must be at least 10 feet in order to accommodate the electric hoist apparatus. Because of the various kinds of apparatus to be installed in the gymnasium, the ceiling height there must also be at least 10 feet.

Some functional areas and functional area elements, for which dimensions were not suggested in Table 3.1, require special consideration as follows below.

Gymnasium

One source has recommended that one-half of the total space occupied by the department should be allocated to the gymnasium (3). This allotment seems high for the general hospital by present day standards. A more realistic allocation of space for the gymnasium may be approximately one-third of the total space.

On the other hand, studies by this author in a general hospital setting, not involved in long-term rehabilitation, indicated that almost two out of every three patients used the gymnasium to some degree during the course of a patient visit. One must presume that this area will be one of high utilization. Essential equipment in even the modestly sized gymnasium consumes considerable space. Therefore, if one has a choice of overestimating space needs, the gymnasium is the logical place to exercise this option.

Patient Waiting Areas

Numerous factors must be considered when attempting to estimate space for patient waiting and holding areas. The amount of space required to accommodate an ambulatory out-patient is less than would be required for a patient in a wheelchair or on a stretcher. One source has suggested that 16 square feet be allocated for the average ambulatory patient and that 25 feet be allowed for wheelchair or litter patients (8). Patton has proposed a formula to satisfy requirements for out-patient waiting areas (15). This formula assumes that the average patient requires 10 square feet of space for seating and suggests the minimum space required for waiting during peak periods.

$$\frac{\text{Number of patient visits per week} \times 10 \text{ square feet} \times \text{number of escorts (usually 1.5 is maximum)}}{\begin{array}{c}5 \text{ days per week} \times \text{number of peak treatment periods} \\ (6 \text{ hourly periods per working day or 3 peak periods} \\ \text{instead of 6 hourly periods})\end{array}} = \begin{array}{l}\text{Space required} \\ \text{for waiting}\end{array}$$

Example:

$$\frac{100 \times 10 \times 1.5}{5 \times 6} = 50 \text{ square feet}$$

In the author's opinion, the problems usually encountered in dealing with out-patient waiting facilities are caused by people accompanying patients to the department rather than patients themselves. If a department is of proper size and operates efficiently, a backlog of patients awaiting treatment seldom occurs. Predicting the number of people who might escort a patient to the department is difficult. If the department's philosophy will be to treat unscheduled out-patients, this factor must also be considered when estimating space requirements for waiting areas.

Underestimating patient and family waiting areas can cause serious operational difficulties as well as produce anxiety and dissatisfaction to patients and staff alike. It is far better to overestimate the space requirements in this area and to make provisions for periods of peak utilization

Storage Facilities

Adequate storage space for equipment, linen, supplies, patient records, and staff needs is essential to the well designed and properly functioning department. The location of these storage areas is also important because of the need to have quick access to those pieces of equipment and supplies that are used routinely. Planning for storage and its location must be done when other space allocations are being considered. The use of alcoves or recessed spaces for wheelchairs, stretchers, and linen carts can be incorporated into the department design and space conserved. Seldom used pieces of equipment might be stored elsewhere in the hospital, thus saving valuable space in the department.

Today, many modular prefabricated storage units are available. These units provide unique flexibility in coping with hospital and departmental storage problems.

Charting Areas

Record keeping has become an increasingly important function of all physical therapy departments. Providing adequate and properly located space for this activity is essential. The charting areas should be close to patient treatment areas. This provides the opportunity for surveillance of patients and still permits the physical therapist to carry out record keeping in satisfactory manner.

A decision to either handwrite or dictate patient evaluation and progress notes must be made early in the planning stages since this may influence space allocations. If progress notes are to be dictated, some privacy is required. This can best be achieved by using glass partitions or screening and sound-proofing by other methods.

Many unique and innovative concepts can be introduced into the charting area (Fig. 3.3). For example, a good feature of any general hospital department is to have a series of treatment timers which correspond to the various treatment rooms within the department. These timers can be easily incorporated into the charting counter.

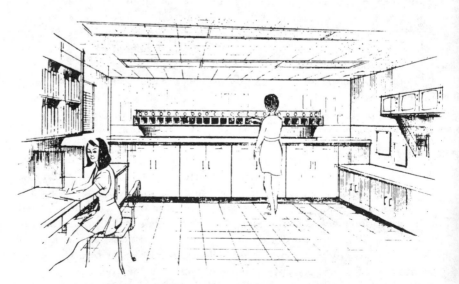

Figure 3.3.   A model charting area with interval treatment timers, dictating booths, T.V. monitors, master annunciator panel and scheduling board.

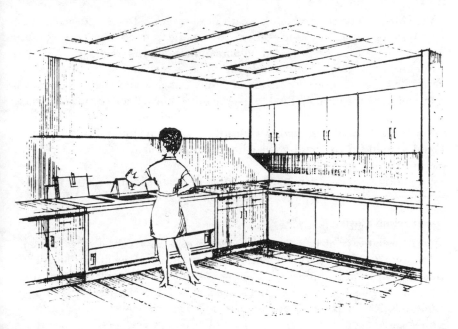

Figure 3.4. A typical work station supporting a treatment cubicle area, with built-in hot packing unit and adequate work space.

Work Stations

Work stations that support specific functional areas within the department are most important and should not be overlooked when space allocations are being considered (Fig. 3.4). The size of each individual work station will depend upon the number of activities to be supported.

If properly located, one work station is usually adequate to support each functional area of the department. When an ideal location is not possible, more than one work station may be required.

Linen Storage and Disposal

Physical therapy departments are among the grestest consumers of linen within the hospital. The need for a ready and adequate source of clean linen is therefore an important consideration. With careful planning, the problems usually encountered with linen storage and disposal can be avoided.

Generally linen is transported to the department from the laundry by special carts. Determine the size of the carts used and provide space in the department for storage of these carts. In this way carts can serve as central sources of clean linen for the department. This also does away with the time-consuming practice of taking linen from a cart and storing it in a linen closet.

The various work stations within the department can be stocked with linen adequate in supply for the needs of the particular areas. In addition, linen storage bins can be constructed beneath most treatment tables. It is mandatory, however, that any linen stored in a patient treatment area not be exposed. Doors must be provided on all cabinets housing linen.

Equally important when considering linen is how it will be disposed of once soiled. Linen chutes located in treatment areas using large amounts of linen would be the ideal method to handle soiled linen. Architectural barriers or cost considerations may make such a system unobtainable. Closed hamper arrangements can be designed as a substitute for linen chutes. Every attempt should be made to avoid using soiled linen hampers which are both unsanitary and unsightly.

Two additional factors will influence the ultimate space needs for the new department and each can have considerable impact on the space allocated.

Construction Costs

Costs are always of paramount importance in any type of construction, and hospitals are no exception. Because hospitals house the ill and incapacitated, every precaution must be taken to ensure safety regardless of expense. Recent technological advances in the mechanical and electrical fields make hospitals safer for patients but tend to increase the costs of construction. Sophisticated signal systems, refined air filtering devices, stand-by electrical plants that begin to function within seconds of electrical failure, and protective measures make hospitals among the most expensive of all structures.

At the present time, hospital costs have been averaging between $100 and $125 a square foot to build, exclusive of land acquisition, architectural fees, equipment, furniture, and site development. The per square foot cost within the structure varies greatly from the cost of storage space, which is the cheapest, to such areas as surgery and radiology, which are the most expensive. The cost of constructing a physical therapy department falls at approximately the average of the over-all hospital cost.

Although hospital costs vary from the small rural one-story structure to the highly sophisticated urban medical center, and from the milder to the more severe climate, these differences are diminishing. With national medical plans and standards becoming more and more common, the rural areas are demanding the same type of health services and facilities available in larger cities.

The constraints imposed by consideration of costs in any construction project can be formidable and will have a bearing on the ultimate amount of space allocated for any hospital department.

Future Expansion

The possibility of future expansion must be considered when estimating space needs. If provisions for expanding the department can be made at the time of original planning, future costs can be reduced significantly and there will be minimal disruption of the service at the time of expansion.

Several things can be done which will enable expansion of the services to occur in an economical and orderly manner. Electrical, plumbing, heating, and cooling systems can be stubbed in. In addition, a wide variety of attractive and functional movable partitions are available today. These partitions provide unique flexibility in already existing departments as well as for future expansion needs.

EQUIPMENT

The various types and amounts of equipment needed for the proposed facility must be considered before preliminary drawings are started. Equipment is classified as either "fixed" or "movable." As the term implies, fixed equipment is either affixed to the building or connected to a service distribution system during construction (14). Some examples of fixed equipment would be stationary hydrotherapy tanks, parallel bars attached to floor surfaces, annunciator systems, etc. Movable equipment will include all those items used in the department which are not fixed or connected to the building such as treatment tables, files, furniture, diathermy, ultrasound machines, etc.

A further classification of fixed equipment is often necessary because of the various options available for dealing with such equipment. It is possible for the contractor to furnish and install the equipment, for the owner to furnish and install the equipment, or for the owner to furnish and the contractor to install the equipment (Table 3.5). The choices among these options must be made known to the architect early in the project so that the cost of construction can be accurately estimated.

A complete equipment check list should be prepared for all required items within the department. The equipment requirements of each functional area within the department should then be listed (Tables 3.6 through 3.9), and cross-checked against the master list. In this way, equipment needs will not be overlooked.

The equipment required for each specific area within the department should be reviewed with the architect on an item by item basis. In this way the architect can determine if space requirements are adequate and if any special installation specifications will be necessary. For example, most of the wall-mounted equipment in the gymnasium will require special wall reinforcement to ensure safe operation. Ceiling moorings with maximum weight potential of 500 pounds may also be necessary in the gymnasium (4). Other equipment may require special consideration in terms of either electrical or plumbing hookups. All reliable equipment manufacturers will have available detailed installation specifications. The physical therapist may have to assist the architect in obtaining this information at an early date.

One must recognize that sufficient equipment is essential to an efficiently operating department. The practice of moving equipment frequently from

Table 3.5
Fixed Equipment Guide and Room Checklist

EXIST	OFCI	OFOI	CFCI	Department	Room	Room No.

CFCI: Contractor Furnished—Contractor Installed
OFOI: Owner Furnished—Owner Installed.
OFCI: Owner Furnished—Contractor Installed

Ceiling Finish:

____accoustical
____gypsum plaster
____Keene's cement plaster
____Portland cement plaster
____height
____reinforced
____color
____other (specify)

Wall Finish:

____gypsum plaster
____Keene's cement plaster
____Portland cement plaster
____drywall
____ceramic tile
____vinyl clad metal
____vinyl
____reinforced
____moisture proof
____color
____other (specify)

Weinscot:

____vinyl
____ceramic tile
____vinyl clad metal
____height
____color
____other (specify)

Base: (1)

____rubber T.S.
____Carpet____
____ceramic tile
____carpet
____color

Floor Finish:

____asphalt tile
____vinyl asbestos   (2)
____sheet vinyl (covered base____)
____ceramic tile
____conductive floor
____terrazzo
____carpet
____sloped to drain
____color
____other (specify)

Doors:

____ ____w × 7' high
____wood
____metal
____lam. plastic
____accordian
____automatic
____swing: in____out____
____color

Curtain Tracks:

____
____
____

Electrical:

____110V receptacle
____220V receptacle
____receptacles, height____
____special locations
____wall clocks
____other (specify)

Plumbing:

____lavatory
____counter sink S (3) D
____service sink (janitor)
____water closet
____urinal
____floor drain
____shower
____drinking fountain
____whirlpool cleaning hose

Communications:

____telephone
____intercom
____public address
____nurse call
____music
____central dictation
____pneumatic tube
____closed circuit T.V.
____T.V. antenna
____annunciator
____other (specify)

Lighting:

____regular indirect
____spotlights
____other (specify)

Miscellaneous:

____mirrors
____clothes hooks
____bulletin boards
____other (specify)

Remarks:
(1) Top Set
(2) Height 4"–6"
(3) Single or Double

Table 3.6
Equipment Check List, Hydrotherapy Area

Description	Room No. or Location	Quantity	Dimen-sions			Fixed	Movable	Model No.	Source of Pur-chase
			W	L	H				
Adjustable Whirlpool Chair (High)									
Adjustable Whirlpool Chair (Low)									
Chair—Regular									
Dressing Cart									
Hubbard Tank									
Hubbard Tank—Adj. Headrest									
Hubbard Tank—Water Stretcher									
Hubbard Tank—Body Hammock									
Hubbard Tank—Electric Hoist									
Hydraulic Patient Lifter									
Infra-Red Generator									
Inside Seat, Arm, Leg, Hip Whirlpool									
Kromayer Lamp									
Linen Hamper									
Lowboy Headrest									
Lowboy Seat									
Mixing Valves									
Mobile Arm, Leg, Hip Whirlpool									
Paraffin Bath									
Ultrasound Generator									
Sitz Bath Chair									
Stationary Arm Whirlpool									
Stationary Arm, Leg, Hip Whirlpool									
Stationary Lowboy Whirl-pool									
Step-up Stool									
Stretcher									
Treatment Table									
Treatment Timer									

one treatment area to another should be discouraged. The abuse to the equipment from constant moving should more than justify purchase of additional units.

At first, it may be difficult to estimate the exact amount of equipment that might be required. If the constraints of the equipment budget are such that only a minimal amount of equipment can be purchased, attempts should be

Table 3.7
Equipment Check List, Treatment Cubicle Area

Description	Room No. or Location	Quantity	Dimensions			Fixed	Movable	Model No.	Source of Purchase
			W	L	H				
Baker									
Cervical Traction Unit									
Chair—Regular									
Chronaximeter									
Colpac Unit									
Dressing Cart									
Electromyograph Unit									
Goniometer									
Hot Pack Unit									
Ice Machine									
Infra-Red Genertor									
Jobst Pressure Unit									
Linen Hamper									
Low Volt Generator									
Medcolator									
Medcosonolator									
Microwave									
Pelvic Traction Unit									
Powder Board									
Rolling Stool									
S.W. Diathermy									
Spirometer									
Step-Up Stool									
TENS Unit									
Treatment Table									
Treatment Timer									
Ultrasound Generator									
Ultraviolet Generator									
X-Ray View Box									

made to establish an equipment contingency fund. This fund would enable the purchase of additional necessary equipment when the department is operational and equipment needs are better known.

Frequently physical therapists have difficulty in obtaining the type of equipment they desire because os cost conscious purchasing agents. This is most unfortunate because the cost savings may later be lost through inefficient or ineffective treatment, frequent repairs, or even disuse. Physical therapists must assert themselves in specifying their equipment needs and not accept unsatisfactory substitutes.

UTILITIES

Utilities are not less important than space and equipment for the efficient and effective operation of the physical therapy department. The physical therapist involved in planning and designing a department will have much to contribute here and should not assume that the architect and others know all about the department's utilities needs.

Electrical Systems

Properly designed electrical systems are essential for the safe and efficient functioning of the department. In addition to the usual and customary requirements of various electrical and building codes other factors must be considered.

Table 3.8
Equipment Check List, Gymnasium Area

Description	Room No. or Location	Quantity	Dimensions			Fixed	Movable	Model No.	Source of Purchase
			W	L	H				
Ankle Exerciser									
Barbell and Rack									
Cane-Adjustable									
Cane-Quad									
Chair-Regular									
Crutches-Axillary (pr.)									
Crutches-Forearm (pr.)									
Cybex									
Disc Weights									
Disc Weight Cart									
Elgin Table									
Finger Ladder									
Gym Mat									
Gym Mat Platform									
Hand Table									
Overhead Pulleys									
Parallel Bars									
Posture Mirror									
Pronator-Supinator Unit									
Quadriceps Table									
Ramp									
Restorator									
Rolling Stool									
Sandbag									
Shoulder Wheel									
Stairs									
Stall Bars									
Standing Bar									
Stationary Bicycle									
Tilt Table									
Treatment Table									
Walker-Adjustable									
Wall Pulleys									
Wrist Roll Unit									

Table 3.9
Equipment Check List, Administrative, and Support Areas

Description	Room No. or Location	Quantity	Dimensions			Fixed	Movable	Model No.	Source of Purchase
			W	L	H				
Annunciator									
Bookcase									
Calculator									
Chair—Conference									
Chair—Desk									
Chair—Secretary									
Chair—Regular									
Conference Table									
Copying Machine									
Desk									
Dictating Equipment									
Filing Cabinet-Letter									
Filing Cabinet-Charts									
Filing Cabinet-Other									
Intercom									
Locker									
Supply Cabinet									
TV Monitor									
Typewriter									
X-Ray View Box									

1. The physical therapist should supply the architect with information on the electrical power requirements of all electrically operated equipment to be used in the department. This information, together with information on the planned location of the equipment, will be helpful in the design of the department's electrical subpanel.

2. Ideally, the electrical subpanel should be located somewhere within the department to facilitate handling any problems related to overloaded circuits.

3. Generally, 110 volt and 220 volt lines will be adequate to handle the equipment needs of the department. The 220 volt power source is usually required for the larger custom built hot pack machines.

4. Any electrically operated equipment to be used within the department must be grounded by means of a three-way plug, and all electrical outlets should receive only the appropriate type of plug.

5. Be generous when planning for electrical outlets. The cost per receptacle is minor when planned for and installed during original construction. The cost is much higher if additional receptacles are installed after construction is completed.

6. The physical therapist must specify the number and location of all electrical outlets. The location of electrical outlets is extremely important, a matter often overlooked in the planing process. Unless otherwise

specified, all outlets will automatically be located 8 to 10 inches above the baseboard. While this is practical for most construction projects, it will present problems in the physical therapy department.

In treatment cubicle areas it is more convenient to have electrical outlets located at a height of 40 inches from the floor. This higher location facilitates plugging and unplugging equipment and does away with unsightly line cords lying on the floor. In addition, the tendency to tip over equipment is reduced and cleaning floor surfaces is made easier.

Certain types of equipment require unusual location of electrical outlets. This pertains to the wall-mounted cervical traction unit, where it is desirable to have the outlet adjacent to the unit. It also applies in the Hubbard tank area where a ceiling locking type outlet must be provided for the hoist motor. The floor outlets for the electrical turbines of the Hubbard tank must be raised from the floor. If properly located, these outlets will be far enough under the tank to permit plugging and unplugging and still not be a hazard to be tripped over.

7. Sources of electricity will also be required in many other areas of the department for dictating equipment, clocks, electric treatment timers, patient call light systems, intercom, piped in music, and specialized equipment such as electrically operated tilt tables, treatment tables, and parallel bars.

Sufficient electrical outlets in the business or receptionist office must also be provided to adequately handle electric typewriters, calculators, etc. Consideration should also be given to the use of floor buffing machines and vacuum cleaners by the janitorial staff.

Plumbing

The plumbing requirements of the physical therapy department are unusual in many respects. Some of the more unique features are listed.

1. A constant source of water pressure and an adequate supply of hot water are essential. The architect must have knowledge of the maximum potential of water in the department. This will require that the architect know the water capacity of all major hydrotherapy equipment. He must then determine if the central source of water and boilers are adequate to sustain the hydrotherapy needs. If not, an independent boiler and water storage tank may be necessary. A maximum temperature of 160° is recommended for hot water in all whirlpool areas.

2. The diameter of all plumbing lines to whirlpools should be ¾ inch. The length of time needed to fill whirlpools will be significantly reduced when using pipes of this diameter.

3. The drainage of hydrotherapy tanks will be expedited by using waste lines of the largest possible diameter. Sometimes it is advantageous to use electrically boosted pumps to speed this process.

4. Sometimes it is possible to cant or tilt hydrotherapy tanks towards the drain. This will assist quick drainage.
5. Floor drains should be provided in all whirlpool and tank areas and the floor sloped slightly to permit adequate drainage of tank overflows.
6. Thermostatic mixing valves are generally recommended for hydrotherapy tanks. The mechanical problems often encountered with these valves makes their value questionable. If independent hot and cold water valves are substituted, make certain these fixtures are easily operated.
7. A water hose for the proper cleaning of all hydrotherapy tanks is necessary. These hoses should be located at the water source on wall surfaces for extremity tanks, but should be overhead and retractable in the Hubbard tank area.
8. Whenever possible, use stainless steel sinks. The chipping and staining of enameled iron with subsequent replacement is more expensive than the original purchase of stainless steel.
9. Sinks are available in all shapes and sizes. The use, whether for hand washing, electrode soaking, general cleaning, etc., will determine the most suitable types. If plaster of paris is to be used in the department, a plaster sink trap should be provided.
10. A source of water supply and drainage is desirable for hot pack machines and mandatory for custom built units.
11. Drinking fountains are required in a variety of areas within the department. Some of these should accommodate wheelchair patients.
12. If a shower is provided, make certain it has adequate room for the disabled patient and that some seating arrangement exists within the shower.
13. The temperature of water in patient restrooms must be kept at safe levels. Plumbing fixtures such as water closets and sinks should be at a height convenient to wheelchair patients. Sinks should extend out well beyond exposed plumbing lines to prevent accidental burns to the lower extremities of wheelchair patients.
14. A mop sink should be provided in the janitor's closet.

Lighting

A variety of approaches are possible for providing high intensity but diffused lighting in the department. Glare should be avoided as much as possible for the benefit of those patients who may be lying supine. Costs usually dictate which method can best be used. Luminous ceiling panels generally produce the best results.

A rheostat located in certain treatment areas, even though expensive, is an ideal way to have control over the intensity of light sources. This would be most advantageous in treatment cubicles.

Certain areas of the department will require additional sources of lighting.

This can be achieved with ceiling spotlights over desks and charting locations, or by the use of special gooseneck lights which pull down from either the wall or the ceiling. These devices can be used when doing electrical muscle testing or wound debridement.

Heating and Cooling

Special attention must be given to the matter of climate control because various environmental conditions exist within the department. Individual room temperature control is the ideal toward which one should strive, but the budget will seldom permit this refinement. Some zone separation must be provided if an acceptable environment is to be achieved. By carefully selecting areas of like function, exposure, and time use, the number of separate zones can be kept to an acceptable minimum.

Although the frequency of air change is important throughout the department, it is imperative in hydrotherapy areas. In these water-laden areas, it is advisable to exhaust the air rather than recirculate it. Throughout the department it is essential that good draft-free air distribution be provided, since in most sections there will be patients who are partially or totally uncovered.

One area of climate control that has not been adequately engineered is in the Hubbard tank or similar full body immersion area. Patients, especially those with burns, experience varying degrees of chilling and discomfort when removed from the tanks. Raising the general room temperature, or using movable infra-red lights, is not the most effective way to remedy this problem.

Supplementary environmental systems could be provided in Hubbard tank rooms. These systems would be similar to the laminar flow systems now used in surgical operating rooms. In that part of the room where the patient would be drying after removal from the Hubbard tank, a portion of the ceiling four feet by eight feet would be dropped to a height of approximately eight feet. The plane of this portion of the ceiling would be finely perforated, and hot air which has been filtered through high efficiency filters would be forced through these small apertures to bathe the patient below (Fig. 3.5). The fan coil unit and filters would be housed above the suspended ceiling. The controls which govern the quantity and temperature of the air desired would be on an adjacent wall, easily accessible to the therapist. This forced air heating unit should overcome some of the discomfort experienced by patients. The unit has been carefully researched and engineered but its effectiveness has not yet been tested in an actual treatment situation.

COMMUNICATION SYSTEMS

A properly conceived and designed system of communications within the physical therapy department will improve overall function immeasurably. There are various communications systems to be considered.

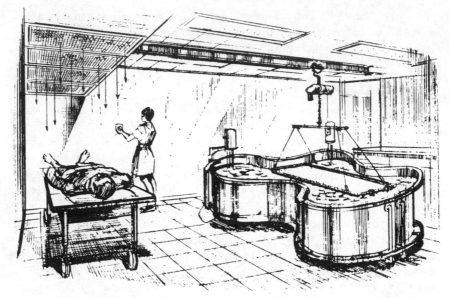

Figure 3.5.   A filtered forced air unit in the Hubbard tank room, with a rheostat on wall to control temperature and flow of air.

Telephones

Primary consideration of telephones must be given to the department's reception or business office area, where a sufficient number of instruments to handle potential demand is necessary. If the department is large, a multitrunk phone installation should be considered. If a great number of outside calls to and from physicians are expected, a direct outside line will be helpful and would not tie up the hospital switchboard. All offices should have phone installations. It is also important to install telephones in the various work areas in the department. This can save staff much time by permitting them to remain in critical work areas and still use the telephones. If telephones are located in various strategic locations throughout the department, they can be used for interdepartmental communications purposes.

Intercoms

Strategically located intercoms can also facilitate the functions of the department. The master control unit is usually located in the main office area, where someone is in attendance at all times. In larger departments, such systems are essential. The disadvantages of having the physical therapy department connected to the main hospital paging system seem to outweigh the advantages. The constant distraction caused by such a system does not seem justifiable for the few pertinent messages that apply to the department during the course of a normal day. The need to contact therapists who may be working in various parts of the hospital seems best served with pocket carried paging units.

Annunciator Systems

One of the most important communications devices required for patient safety and efficient department operations is an annunicator system (Fig. 3.6). This system can be designed in a variety of ways and can include several features. The major function to be served by such a system is to provide a patient the opportunity to signal that he requires assistance. A call button, which a patient can activate, is essential. Once the call button has been activated, some means, either auidble, visual, or both, is necessary so that the signal source can be easily identified. This can be accomplished by a master panel which should be located in an area easily visible by staff. The central charting area and the main secretarial office are usually the best locations. Dome lights over each treatment area are also recommended for quick identification of a signal source. This would make it possible to ascertain the source of a signal when the master panel cannot be seen.

Another desirable feature of an annunciator system is for it to have the capability of determining occupancy of patient treatment areas. Each treatment area of the department should have a corresponding position on the master panel. When a patient is placed in a treatment room, a toggle switch is turned on which activates a light corresponding to that room on the master panel. When this light is on, staff is immediately aware that the particular

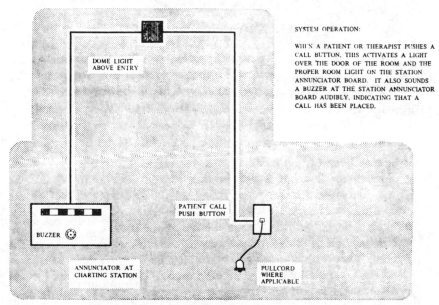

Figure 3.6. Components of an annunciator system.

treatment area is occupied and unavailable for use. This will conserve considerable staff time in searching for an available treatment location for waiting patients.

As suggested, many variations are possible when designing an annunciator system, and for the most part, these will depend on the size of the facility and cost considerations. Cost should not be a major consideration, even when high, since patient safety is the primary concern.

Pneumatic Tube Station

Pneumatic tubes can be used for transmitting certain materials and communications throughout the hospital. The location of the receiving and sending stations should be in a convenient area, preferably within the main secretarial office of the department.

Closed Circuit Television

Still another dimension of patient safety and improved function of the department can be provided through television monitoring. It is often desirable to have the ability to monitor patients receiving treatment in certain areas, such as the Hubbard tank room, whirlpool areas, and the gymnasium. The monitoring station should be located within an area staffed at all times. The cost considerations to install such systems are not usually expensive. There is sufficient justification for closed circuit television in even an average size department.

FLOOR SURFACES

Safety, durability, and ease of maintenance are factors to consider when choosing a floor surface. Several different options are available and those used will depend to some degree upon cost and type of floor surfaces used elsewhere within the hospital. The nonskid waxes commercially available today make the use of vinyl and vinyl asbestos floor covering quite safe.

In hydrotherapy units, vinyl sheeting, terrazzo, and ceramic tile can all be used to good advantage. Terrazzo-like floor surfaces in these areas seem to have the most advantage, since they resist water, are easily maintained, and are possibly less noisy than ceramic tile. Ceramic tile floor surfaces are more difficult to maintain.

In all other areas of the department, vinyl asbestos or pure vinyl tile or vinyl sheeting can be used with considerable success. The advantages of using some of the newer vinyl sheetings is that they can be coved at the baseboard. This coving provides a good appearance and is easy to maintain.

Carpeting is becoming increasingly more commonplace in many areas of hospitals. There are certain advantages to using carpeting in the department. It is less fatiguing to workers, quieter, and as easily maintained as other floor surfaces. A carpeted surface would pose obvious disadvantages in the hydrotherapy area and on the floor within the parallel bars. Perhaps less obvious are the difficulties carpeting poses to patients who propel their own wheelchairs, and the potential hazards it poses to ambulating patients who have certain gait deviations such as toe-drag or toe-scuff. Decisions of whether to install carpeting and where should be weighed with care.

DECOR

An intelligently designed department can be greatly complemented by tasteful decor. The imaginative use of color and furnishings can lend a pleasant atmosphere for patients and staff alike.

Durable and easily maintained vinyl wall fabrics are available in a variety of colors and textures. It has been suggested that colors that are stimulating may be desirable in exercise areas. Pastel tones of cool colors such as green, blue, and violet are considered restful (4). In most hospital construction projects, the services of an interior decorating firm are retained. Consultation with such decorating firms will assist the physical therapist in achieving an unusual yet coordinated decorative scheme.

Every attempt should be made to envision areas where potential abuse to wall surfaces or corners might occur. These areas should be protected by the use of corner guards or strip-like protection materials on wall surfaces.

ARCHITECTURAL DRAWINGS

Preliminary Drawings

The architect will be ready to start the preliminary drawings when the schematic drawings have been reviewed and approved. Unlike a schematic drawing, where dimensions are only approximate (see Fig. 3.1), a preliminary drawing requires accurate dimensions of the various components to be included in the department. One must be prepared to make several compromises at this stage because it is unusual to obtain all that is desired within a fixed space allocation. Priorities for essential services and optimal department operation must be established. If trade-offs must be made, make certain that essential services are not sacrificed.

When the preliminary drawings are started, the architect must be aware of every piece of equipment, fixed or movable, that will be required as well as all cabinet work, plumbing fixtures, furniture, and anything else that will occupy floor space.

In most instances, the first preliminary plan will be the total responsibility of the architect. If the physical therapist has formulated thoughts on how the department should be designed, he should communicate these ideas to the architect either verbally or graphically. In fact, this may be done before the schematic drawings are stated.

The importance of the physical therapist becoming involved in preliminary drawings should not be underestimated, even if particular skills in this area are meager. The value of conjointly working on this phase of planning will produce preliminary plans that more accurately reflect the wishes of the therapist and still remain architecturally feasible. In addition, the number of conferences and revisions usually required with regard to preliminary drawings will be reduced.

The architect can provide the physical therapist with sufficient information to enable the therapist to carry out some preliminary drawings. This information should include the location of the department, the overall dimensions, the location of architectural obstructions, stairwells, and elevators, the physical relationship of the department to other departments, and any other special considerations that might influence the floor plan.

If it is possible to have an influence on the dimensions and shape of the space to be provided, this could markedly ease the design process. Areas that are too long and narrow or turn too many corners present serious design problems and will impede layout and function. A space that approaches a rectangle is generally more desirable. Structural columns have an affinity for appearing in the most undesirable locations. Know as soon as possible where these columns will be located in order to design around them or to incorporate them into the department design in an unobtrusive manner. It is also possible to have the columns serve some useful purpose. Usable wall space, especially in the gymnasium, is another important factor to consider when making preliminary drawings.

There are several ways one can go about preparing preliminary drawings or floor plans. Recognize that it is not unusual to go through this process several times before arriving at what might seem an ideal floor plan.

A satisfactory method to work on floor plans can be achieved by cutting out to scale from construction paper the various desired components to be included in the department. It is usually easier to work with large scale measurements, such as one-quarter inch or one-half inch to the foot. Several attempts at rearranging these cut-outs will be necessary to obtain a workable plan. One should attempt to group all or most activities requiring plumbing as close together as possible. The cost savings is substantial if this can be accomplished.

Even after arriving at what might seem a workable floor plan, different approaches should be attempted. It is also advantageous to review these plans with other physical therapists whenever possible. These rough preliminary lay-outs are then transmitted to the architect who will have ideas of his own, independently gathered, which will complement the ultimate design of the department.

It is imperative to study and restudy the plan several times at this stage of development. Check all room sizes and their accessways. Make certain that equipment will fit into the designed areas. Door widths and heights are critical in several areas of the department. Scale models of wheelchairs and stretchers can be used to check if accessways and door widths are of proper size. Most construction and fire regulations require a minimum corridor width of eight feet. Door widths of 46 inches off of an eight-foot corridor will accommodate a wheeled stretcher. In areas where two-way traffic is anticipated, door widths should be at least four feet.

It is advantageous to eliminate the use of cubicle curtains whenever possible. These curtains may offer flexibility but they do not provide privacy and they are not aesthetically pleasing. Vinyl fabric accordion doors can be substituted for cubicle curtains with great success. When used as the front portion of a treatment cubicle, these accordion doors should open to a minimum width of 46 inches.

The purpose of the very careful review at this stage of planning is that changes are expected. This is not the case when working drawings have been bid or construction started.

Working Drawings

Working drawings consist of a series of drawings that describe in great detail the floor plan and the major systems such as plumbing, lighting scheme, elevations or drawings of critical areas, and heating and cooling systems. All fixed equipment is usually depicted in the detailed floor plan.

A variety of symbols is used in the preparation of working drawings to depict elements of electrical, plumbing, communications, heating, cooling and other systems within the department. A list of the more commonly used symbols is provided as a reference source (Fig. 3.7).

At this stage it is helpful to have an accurate method to review each area of the department to ensure that all items have been included. The room checklist shown in Table 3.5 can be used to review each area of the department on an item-by-item basis. This same checklist is also useful after construction has started.

In the preparation of working drawings, the architect must reflect every minute detail of the plan. The contractor will bid the construction project from these detailed working drawings. His cost estimates will be based on what the working drawings and specifications require. Bidding on any construction project is usually a very competitive process and cost estimates must be adhered to closely. Any changes proposed by a client after construction has started must usually be assumed by the client. These changes generally are quite costly and should be avoided if possible.

CONSTRUCTION

Once the actual construction project is started, the physical therapist should be readily available for consultation with the architect and the

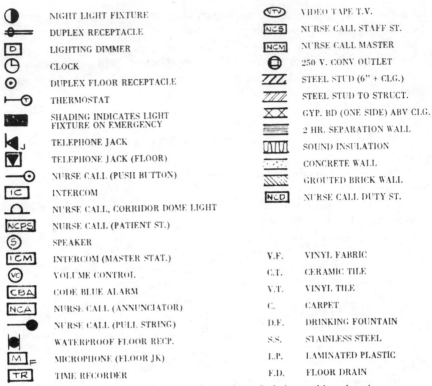

Figure 3.7. A list of commonly used symbols in working drawings.

contractor. It is not desirable, at least in the opinion of the contractor, to be underfoot while actual construction is under way. Nevertheless, it is advisable to review the work in progress at periodic intervals to make certain that all elements of the plan are being fulfilled. Errors of omission and misinterpretations of working drawings are not unusual. Bringing these matters to the attention of the contractor will prevent unnecessary delays in the construction project. The use of the room checklist previously discussed (Table 3.5) will provide a systematic method to review the various stages of the construction project.

The availability of the physical therapist when fixed equipment is being installed is critical, because variations of a few inches in some equipment installation can pose serious operational problems. The proper operation of all systems and fixed equipment will be guaranteed by the contractor, but it is more desirable to make any necessary adjustments or corrections prior to the opening of the department.

CONCLUSIONS

The important aspects of planning and designing a physical therapy department for the general hospital setting have been reviewed. The concepts suggested have applicability to all settings where physical therapy services are provided.

No attempt has been made to suggest "model plans" for general hospitals of any size. Rather, basic concepts of planning and design have been discussed in detail. Physical therapy departments must be planned and designed to meet the demands and requirements of individual hospital progrms. Stereotyped plans should be discouraged, since they can act as constraints to the various approaches of delivering physical therapy services.

The physical therapist has the opportunity to provide the necessary direction and consultation for department planning and design. The material in this text is offered as a guideline to those involved in the planning and design of physical therapy departments.

The entire process from start to finish is challenging and demanding. The results of these efforts will be rewarding when the project has been completed and ideas have been translated into a well designed department.

Acknowledgment. The author wishes to acknowledge the help of the architectural firm of Harnish, Morgan and Causey, Ontario, California, in preparing the figures and advising on the architectural considerations in this chapter. The information and data supplied by colleagues within and outside the profession is also gratefully acknowledged.

References

1. American Hospital Association: *Estimating Space Needs and Cost in General Hospital Construction.* American Hospital Association, Chicago, 1963.
2. American Hospital Association: *Hospital Statistics*, 1979 Edition. American Hospital Association, Chicago, 1979.
3. American Hospital Association: *Physical Therapy—Essentials of a Hospital Department.* American Hospital Association, Chicago, 1960.
4. American Hospital Association: *Physical Therapy Service—A Guide to Organization and Management.* American Hospital Association, Chicago, 1965.
5. Burton, L.G.: Planning the physical therapy department—Construction program for rehabilitation facilities and services. J. Am. Phys. Ther. Assoc., 45: 1154–1157, 1965.
6. California Administrative Code: Title 22, Section 70561 (register 75 No. 24, 6-14-75).
7. Cardenas, A.F., Dicus, R.G., Magistro, C.M., and McKillip, J.B.: *Physical Therapy Productivity Measurements—Report of a Pilot Study Project* (unpublished). Supported by a grant from the Physical Therapy Fund, Inc., and on file with the Foundation for Physical Therapy, Inc., Washington, 1974.
8. Doctor, R.L.: Personal communication. U.S. Reynolds Army Hospital, Fort Sill, Oklahoma, 1973.
9. Doctor, R., Reardon, J., and Woodard, C.: Personal communication. Tri-Service Physical Therapy Committee, 1973.
10. Fredrickson, D.: Space and program development. Phys. Ther., 50: 1179–1186, 1970.
11. Heath, J.L.: Personal communication. Naval Regional Medical Center, Oakland, California, 1973.
12. Joint Commission on Accreditation of Hospitals: *Accreditation Manual for Hospitals*, 1981 Edition. Joint Commission on Accreditation of Hospitals, Chicago, 1980.
13. Magistor, C.M., and Harnish, J.D.: Planning the physical therapy department—Design and construction. J. Am. Phys. Ther. Assoc., 45: 1158–1162, 1965.
14. Mooney, L.P.: Construction guideline for physical therapy departments. J. Am. Phys. Ther. Assoc., 50: 349–353, 1970.
15. Patton, F.L.: Planning the physical therapy department—Justification and general cost of space. J. Am. Phys. Assoc. 45: 1165–1169, 1965.
16. Study of health facilities construction costs: A report to the Congress of the United States by the Comptroller General, 1972.

17. Taylor, E.: Personal communication. Hospital Administrative Services, American Hospital Association, Chicago, Illinois, 1980.
18. United States of America Standards Institute: *American Standards Specifications for Making Buildings and Facilities Accessible to, and Usable by, the Physically Handicapped.* Standard No. A-117.1. United States of America Standards Institute, New York, 1961.
19. Wright, B.W.: Health care planning—Acts, agencies, and activities of the federal government. Phys. Ther., *60:* 1017–1021, 1980.

chapter 4

RECORDS

Henry C. Wessman

In athletics, the team "puts it all together" to break records. In health care, the records "put it all together" to solidify the team. The purpose of this chapter on Records is to "put *it* all together" by a comprehensive review and updating of uses, requirements, principles, and types.

Records in the physical therapy department have historically been considered to be in one of two categories; clinical or administrative (7, 21). Clinical records, such as referrals and progress notes, are related directly to patient care. Administrative records, such as departmental statistics and records, are not related directly to patient care, but are no less important than clinical records.

Record keeping, a frequently disdained chore in physical therapy, is much too important to pass over lightly. As noted by Carlin, the existence of accurate, meaningful methods of recording factual material is one of the most significant attributes of a scientific profession (21).

USES AND REQUIREMENTS

The inevitable cannot be escaped—records must be kept. Logic dictates the necessity of maintaining good records in physical therapy, if for no other reason than to serve as a control of operations (7). But there are many more reasons. Some of the reasons pertain to expanding the potential for physical therapy as a "front-line" health care profession.

Because physical therapists minister to the health care needs of the individual, betterment of patient care must be considered as the primary purpose for record keeping. All other purposes are secondary (89, 109).

Communication

The apparent dichotomy between specialization of care and the team approach increases the need for medical records to serve as a means of communication among clinicians. The effectiveness of the team approach for comprehensive patient care requires accurate, efficient patient care records (13). These records communicate best if they are standardized (8, 33). In a rapidly changing environment, such as an acute care hospital, records must be kept up to date so that the patient care will be consistent with the patient's needs. In situations such as this, the multidisciplinary progress notes have their greatest impact (11, 29, 77, 104). Forkner points out the need for greater communication of the patient's medical information because of the high mobility of our society (40). Finally, the carefully documented departmental record must be the vital transmission link subserving all other purposes for records.

Quality of Care Assessment

Related closely to effective communication is the use of feedback in the assessment of the quality of care. A critical review of departmental administrative records should display strengths or weaknesses within the department. Inquiry is the basis of scientific endeavor. Uncovered deficiencies should be considered as possible topics for inservice education (12, 16). The review of quality is generally equated with peer review. It is important to note that staff personnel should be made aware of the criteria upon which they are being judged (61, 85). Specifically, the criteria of thoroughness, reliability, analytically sound logic, and efficiency should be considered when assessing quality of care (88).

When reviewing clinical records for the purpose of assessing quality of care, the standards used must be standards of care rather than standards of the process of care (37). The review should not be for the sake of the record. A valid audit must also include a measurement of the outcome of the patient's treatment (92), and in some manner, a measurement of the patient's satisfaction with his management. Quality factors should include patient safety, care documentation, and comfort (41). As Graves (49) points out, quality is not quantity; but as we continually refer to something in terms of quality, it, with time, begins to have quantity and more objective criteria associated with its assessment. The clinical record is such an entity. In fact, one of the primary purposes of the problem-oriented medical record is to provide that all-important "feedback loop" for assessment of treatment regimen. Weed et al. refer to the "short loop" and "long loop" systems (103). The "short loop" audit is responsive to the point of preventing mistakes in patient care. The "long loop" audit can be used to improve systemwide and/or individual practitioner performance. \

Education

Departmental records should serve as an educational resource for the departmental staff; students; the profession, fellow health team members, including the patient, physician, administrator, and other workers; and the public (104).

Staff education is an essential part of physical therapy (82). To be effective, this education should relate directly to current problem areas that physical therapists have identified in the clinic. Mature professionals learn most efficiently and effectively in a problem-solving setting (16). Continuing education should include documentation of active learner participation, ready feedback, content relative to current clinical problems, and incentives that relate the task directly to the goal, i.e., solving the problem (16). The primary goal in using records for staff education should be to develop the most basic of clinical resources, the ability of individual therapists to learn and think on their own (94). One method of doing this, as discussed by Dreyfus et al. (30), is to conduct periodic "problem audits" within the department. These audits amount to a type of peer review which is of great value in continuing education. One other method of using the record as a continuing education tool is to involve selected staff members in organized continuing education courses, such as those produced by the American Physical Therapy Association and its components. Staff members who attend these courses should be expected to return to their clinical setting and examine the current patient care practices by review of the department's clinical records relating to the topics of the courses. In this manner, the entire staff will benefit from organized continuing education programs.

Departmental records should serve as the interface for the student as he relates didactic coursework to early and extended clinical affiliation. Written documentation of the activities in the clinic will allow the student rapid assimilation into the clinical milieu. Also, documentation of patient care by the student will allow the clinical supervisor an opportunity to determine the progress of the student. Although neither the quality nor the quantity of recorded data may be particularly related to the outcome of patient care (37), audit of the student's written reports, coupled with patient response, will allow the clinical supervisor to assess the student's level of function.

Departmental records serve as a source of education and information for other health team workers (109). Properly written and documented, the information that emanates from within the department can be used to "teach" the physician, administrator, and other workers the value and productivity of physical therapy. One other health team member who can learn from documentation in the department is the patient. Pascasio (82), Dinsdale et al. (29), and Weed (103–107), have all noted the value of including the patient as a member of the decision-making process in the clinical setting. With this team emphasis, education of the patient is not only desirable, it is absolutely essential. This is particularly true in light of the comparatively low compliance to regimen noted for home programs in physical therapy (72). Patient education and compliance can be improved if some ingenuity, such as that noted by Magill (70) is used in preparing home instruction programs.

Public education, be it called public relations, consumerism, consumer relations, or public information, is an essential purpose of documenting activities within the physical therapy department. Documentation must precede any attempt to present a positive profile of physical therapy to the community. Well planned, carefully documented studies can have the added benefit of reiterating the value of the restorative services offered by physical therapy in particular, and rehabilitation in general (62, 108).

Research

As noted by Carlin (21), original clinical research and investigation must be continually developed as the basis for clinical practice in physical therapy. Two hallmarks of a profession are self-evident: the ability to perform from a firm scientific base, and the ability to control professional destiny through documentation and research of prior accomplishments. Scientific methods must be carried into clinical practice. Gordon notes that anyone who has attempted a serious piece of clinical research will recognize the limitations and frustrations of current medical documentation (48). Standardized, consistently kept records are of great value in retrospective clinical studies and provide the information base out of which questions for prospective studies arise.

Organizational procedures for facilitating research in the physical therapy department have been described (32), as have strategies for integrating the research process into daily clinical practice (47). The literature in physical therapy now contains pertinent resources on research methods, from the "quick and easy" (25) to the more complex (23). Techniques for locating, filing and retrieving scientific information, such as those discussed by Lehmkuhl (67), are adaptable to the clinic. Implementation of interaction with computer personnel is also of benefit to the development of ongoing clinical research activities in physical therapy (112).

Motivation

Records documented in the department should serve as a reinforcement tool for staff personnel. Equally important, in our settings where patient participation is essential, is the use of documented patient activity as a motivational tool (78). Documented feedback to the patient in the form of graphic or recorded information can be a powerful tool in operant conditioning or behavior modification, providing the information is related to reinforcement of the desired behavior and coupled with proper reward (72).

Administrative Control

Efficient and effective clinical practice is based on the application of sound administrative principles (52, 69). These principles, in turn, are based on accurate documentation. Such factors as cost analysis in budgeting, staff and patient time scheduling, standards of care, and future planning must have a sound data base. Although quality care (97) and future growth cannot be legislated or guaranteed by data gathering requirements, intelligent use of documentation is fundamental to both of these sought after entities. Without documentation, the excellent administrative studies of Burton et al. (19), Gee and Hickok (43–45), Patton (84), and Price (91), could not have been possible. Employee satisfaction, and equality, can be achieved only when an accurate, standardized, and uniform performance appraisal is applied to all employees (52).

Medical Legal Aspects

It has been estimated that physicians spend approximately 13 percent of their professional time in record keeping (97). Much of this high cost of time is due to the assumed legality of the record—a sort of forensic defense mechanism. This attitude is also prevalent in the allied health fields. Confidentiality, which at one time was between the patient and the physician, is now between the patient and the hospital team (1). This increased level of responsibility, accepted rightfully by the professional allied health worker, bears directly on the quality of thought and documentation that the worker places in the hospital record. All such documentation should of course be thorough, accurate, dated, and signed.

The relationship of the physical therapist assistant to the written record is unclear. In some areas of record keeping, such as in nursing, the assistant's counterpart takes an active role in "charting." In still others, such as in the notes of the physician's assistant, cosignature by the physician-in-charge is required. At the present time, the general consensus is that cosignature by the physical therapist should be included with any medical record entries made by the physical therapist assistant. This places the responsibility for action of the assistant directly on the therapist, and gives both the maximum legal protection. Obviously, the regulations concerning records kept by assistants will vary from state to state and in accord with changing federal regulations concerning health care.

Third Party Requirements

As a result of the evolution of payment methods for health care, documentation for the purpose of receiving payment is a major concern in the physical therapy department (63). Although as much as 20 percent of the data required by third parties may be unnecessary (97), the hard fact is that the record must be completed for payment. There is a need to create more realistic requirements in regard to the information necessary for third-party payers. In the meantime, the clinician has the obligation to present a factual, positive documentation of his or her activities. This is particularly true in the progress noted of chronic cases, where third-party payers expect professional attitudes, care, and documentation. Most insurance carriers have no intention of paying professional costs when the documentation implies custodial care.

Societal Benefits

The connection between daily documentation in the clinic and general humanitarian benefits may be difficult to comprehend. Acheson has pointed out that the advancement of knowledge as a result of the cumulative effect of medical documentation has a profound effect in treatment and cure of various disease processes (1). This, coupled with the educational and administrative functions of records, makes the patient, you, and society the beneficiaries of scientific record keeping.

PRINCIPLES

The previous section addressed the primary principle of record keeping: there must be a reason for the record. This section addresses other important principles of records and record keeping.

Function and Purpose

Anderson (7) notes that the function of any record form in physical therapy may be to notify, order, claim, report, acknowledge, certify, or agree. The combination of any one of these functions with a specified use or requirement, as identified in the foregoing section, should produce a clear purpose for any record that is to be kept.

Communicability

The content of any record must be communicable—capable of being transmitted and understood—if its function and purpose are to be fulfilled. The record must be characterized by accuracy, brevity, clarity, objectivity, and specificity (21, 109). The record must also be legible and identifiable, both in terms of the initiator and the recipient. Abbreviations, initials, and codes should not be used unless there is an available key which has been approved by the institution for inclusion in the medical record. The terminology used must be understandable and devoid of ambiguity, jargon, and verbosity. In a study of terms used in medical records, Gordon found approximately 24,000 different terms used to name 3,700 to 3,800 specific diseases (48). The rest of the terms were synonyms or descriptors. Preciseness and specificity of terms are basic requirements in medical recording. When these are practiced consistently, the size of the medical record may be reduced by 60 to 80 percent or more (48). In our present society, speed of communication must also be an inherent characteristic of the record. This can be accomplished partly by the use of multipart forms (3). Such forms also conserve labor and avoid errors. Speed can also be enhanced by the use of dictation equipment (97), and by electronic processing of data from all types of departmental records (81, 93, 95, 111).

Standardization

Standardization is a means for achieving consistency. Consistency in record keeping is essential for making reliable comparisons, e.g., in comparing discharge status with admission status, or in comparing the average daily number of patient visits in January with the average in July. Standardization and consistency are necessary for any multi-institutional project such as that described by Savander (92).

As record processing becomes more highly automated, standardization of data input will become necessary (33). This will be true of both administrative and clinical record material. Whereas the care given patients in physical therapy will always remain highly individualized, the input language and data concerning each patient will have to be standardized for processing (6, 8, 105, 106). One of the current basic problems with medical records is the lack of structure and rules regarding the recording and organization of the information in the records (33). It may be well to interject here that educators have the task of teaching students how to deal with clinical facts in a thorough, reliable, and analytically sound manner (94). Even in the area of record keeping, the teaching should be a core of behavior and analytical inquiry, rather than isolated facts concerning records. The Weed system teaches such an organized approach to the medical record (104). In this system, the clinician is instructed to organize the data around each problem of the patient. The resultant problem list becomes a dynamic table of contents for the patient's record. The problem-oriented medical record (POMR) goes a long way toward structuring and standardizing the patient record (104). As noted by Feitelberg (35), the POMR is a system—adherance to the rules of the system sets a standard that can be measured. A non-system is not standardized, and cannot be audited. Standardization of terminology of problem titles, such as that conducted by the Department of Physical Medicine at the University of Minnesota Medical School (51), carries this concept one step closer to computerization. Computerization requires standardization.

Form Development and Design

Development and design of a new record form should be undertaken only after careful analysis of need, and careful review of existing forms to prevent duplication and to keep unused space on record forms to a minimum. A new form should not be developed and designed unless there is ample justification for its existence. A rubber stamp can be used to imprint a new item on an already existent form (78, 101). Research indicates that as much as 50 percent of the paper surface in many medical records forms goes unused (3). Storing and microfilming blank paper is expensive and unnecessary.

Staff assistance in development of a new form will enhance ultimate staff acceptance (7). Other services that may be involved with the form, such as data processing and medical records, should be consulted in its development and design.

All forms should be part of a master numbering system (3, 7), which is essential for identification and good control of supply. The master numbering system should include a copy of each form and a statement of title, number, subject, purpose, and principal user (3). Other principles for form development are (3, 7, 53, 79):

1. Carefully scrutinize the proposed form to determine the need and purpose for every item of information asked on the form. Consider information needed for anticipated clinical research.
2. Use clear, understandable, and objective words and phrases on the form, and provide clear-cut directions for completing the form.
3. Whenever possible use terminology in the item headings that is consistent for all the record forms in the hospital.
4. Consider how the form will be used to depict change (if that is one of its purposes), i.e., whether change will be shown by repeated use of one copy or by use of multiple copies of the form.

The principles of form design reflect back on the function and purpose of the particular form. The following principles are important in the design of forms for physical therapy (3, 7, 21, 53, 79):

1. Assure overall uniformity and standardization of:
   a. Paper size, binding edge, and margin.
   b. Quality of paper: this will be dependent on the expected life of the form.
   c. Size and color of printing: for maximum legibility, black print on white paper is preferred. Gray or brown ink will give emphasis to hand-written or typewritten entries.
   d. Spacing: dependent on intended use for typewritten or hand-written entry.
2. Avoid the use of colored forms because of occasional difficulty in photocopying or microfilming. A colored edge may be used for identification.
3. Use multipart forms whenever possible.
4. Design the form with the intent of conserving time for completion. Provide a logical sequence of items (such as date of birth then age) for ease of entry.
5. Include standard items and information on the form, e.g., designated spaces for identity of patient and dates of entries, name of hospital or agency, and date of initiation or revision of form; and locate the standard items and information in standard places on the form to be consistent with all other forms.
6. Edit the form carefully before it is printed.

The principles of form development and design described above can of course be used in reviewing and revising a department's existing forms.

Location

The principle of proper location of the record dictates that administrative or statistical records be retained within the department (21). Clinical records should ideally be available at any terminal within the hospital where medical care is given to the particular patient in question. Because our communication network is not yet that sophisticated, however, the key records are kept where they will be used. This is appropriate because, as Acheson notes (1), the usefulness of medical information in patient care falls off rapidly with time. Patient care records are "needed when they are needed." In a recent study on problems with medical records of ambulatory patients, Tufo and Speidel noted that the major difficulties were the unavailability of the record and the lack of inclusion of latest reports (99). In physical therapy, the implication is that the treatment records should be maintained in the department (3). This presupposes that adequate progress noted and results of evaluative procedures will be forwarded to the hospital chart or referring physician as soon as they are available. A patient file card will allow rapid review of current treatment (7). In a hospital setting, the total clinical records should be incorporated into the patient's chart when treatment is discontinued. In a setting other than a hospital, the record should be retained with an appropriate summary forwarded to the referring physician.

Ownership and Retention

In the hospital setting, all records, both administrative and clinical, are the property of the hospital (3). Information on the clinical record cannot be released without the consent of the patient or his agent (3). This principle must be kept in mind when conducting clinical research (1, 56). A schedule for disposition of departmental records should be established based on experience, needs, and relevant state statutes (3). The length of time that medical records are retained and the form of retention is controversial. Inpatient records which have clinical or scientific potential are usually retained for a period of 25 years after discharge or death (3). In certain institutions where the use of medical records for scientific purposes is limited, a ten-year retention period is considered to be the desired minimum (3). In both instances, it is desirable to retain a summary card showing the name of the physician, diagnoses, and other pertinent data prior to destruction of the record (3).

PATIENT CARE RECORDS

Referrals

The referral form may run the gamut from a signed prescription blank completed in the physician's office to the highly structured modality check list. Both of these types of referral have advantages and disadvantages. The real key to the successful referral relationship is when the physician identifies the reasons or goals to be considered in physical therapy, and the treatment plan is then completed in an air of mutual agreement with the physical therapist and the patient. Ultimately, the referral form must be signed and dated by the referring physician (4). Other items that should be readily available include: name of patient, patient's address, room number if an inpatient, patient's birth date, sex, referral service, insurance or Medicare number, and working diagnosis. Some indication of the number and frequency of treatments desired and the mutually agreed upon date of recheck should also be available. Any special precautions or special instructions should be available to the physical therapist. Inpatient and outpatient referral forms should be standardized within the hospital, and within the entire community, for ease of completion. The referral mechanism is essentially the same for the various settings in which physical therapists practice. The mode may be different depending on the clients served (2, 4, 58, 59, 61, 65, 71).

Evaluation Forms

There might be almost as many evaluation forms as there are physical therapists. Certainly, there are as many evaluation forms as there are kinds of evaluations. The true number lies somewhere in between because each facility has its own adaptations of the forms for tests and measurements. A few items should be included on each evaluation form. These items are: patient identification, the date of the evaluation, and the signature of the therapist conducting the test. In addition, Carlin advocates that each form should have a key for interpretation of the data (21). She notes that an incomplete key or subjective recording leads invariably to erroneous interpretation. From her review of abuses come the principles of factual assessment and recording, ready identification, keyed interpretation, and consistency in the performance of evaluative procedures (21).

Generating a complete list of all evaluation forms used in physical therapy is impossible, and would be quite beyond the scope of this chapter and this book. The variety of evaluation forms reflects the variety of evaluations, tests, and measurements used in physical therapy. The full variety of forms and methods is well represented under the category of "Tests and Measurements" in the published indexes to the official journal of the American Physical Therapy Association (5, 64); under the same category and under "Evaluation" in the annual subject index published each December in that journal; in the special features "Abstracts of Current Literature" and "Book Reviews" published monthly in the same journal; and even in the advertisements of book publishers. Some evaluation forms are available directly from manufacturers of equipment used in physical therapy (34, 98). In addition, professional colleagues in other settings are often most generous in their willingness to share the evaluation forms that they use (2, 51, 58, 65, 71).

Because many physical therapy departments and individual therapists devise or adapt evaluation methods and forms for their own use, the theory and logical requirements of measurement are important principles to be considered (23, pp. 7–83; 50). These principles have much to do with the reliability of measurement or evaluation, the kinds of data obtained, and what can be done (and what cannot be done) with the data.

Specialized Forms

Medicare certification and plan forms are available commercially (14, 90). These forms, and other forms related to Medicare and Medicaid, may be available through the fiscal intermediary. The outpatient appointment card is an important specialized form (7). This card should include the patient's name, day and hour of treatment, and signature of the person making the appointment. Physical therapy departments that conduct or participate in clinical research must be concerned with forms for obtaining the informed consent of patients who participate as subjects in the research (23, p. 322).

Progress Notes

Progress notes are the building blocks of clinical physical therapy (109). Improvement of patient care is the most important function of progress notes. Communication through progress notes allows members of all health services to know what the patient is accomplishing in each given area. Medical legal aspects of progress notes cannot be too strongly emphasized. If the note is a carefully observed and factually recorded entry, it is of utmost value in any legal action that may be taken. Progress notes must be objective. All observations and recordings must be the result of tangible tests or measurements. If this is not possible, lead sentences such as "The patient appears to . . . " or "The patient states . . . " should be used. Patient attitude and mental condition are best expressed in this manner. Objective progress notes are also of great value in education and research.

The progress note should contain patient identification, date, and signature of therapist. Progress notes should be written when 1) the patient is initially treated, 2) the patient's condition changes during the course of treatment, and 3) the patient is discharged (109). The initial note should be written the first day of treatment and should contain the physical therapist's objective evaluation of the patient. The note should include the diagnosis, proposed treatment plan, and location and severity of the involvement. Any unusual condition should be examined and recorded. When appropriate, muscle strength, joint range of motion, and general functional level should also be recorded. Both the involved and contralateral areas should be measured for comparison and future reference. The patient's reaction to the initial treatment should be recorded. If the patient is being readmitted, the initial note should be specific as to the reason.

The notes written during the course of patient care should tell the complete clinical story of the patient from admission to discharge (109). Notes should be written whenever there is a change in the treatment plan, or when there is a change in the mental attitude toward treatment or disability. Regression as well as progression should be noted. Exact positioning and equipment used should be reported. The temperature or setting modalities should be recorded. The length of treatment time and required rest periods are pertinent observations to record. Appliances ordered, the date of application and termination, and the exact placement on the patient should be recorded. Periodic assessment of the patient's level of understanding or the education that the patient is receiving should also be recorded.

The frequency of entry of the running progress note is determined by the condition of the patient and departmental policy. The more chronic the patient, the less frequent the notes need appear. Many departments specify that notes must be written at given intervals (59), such as prior to rounds. Caldwell describes a suspense file which alerts the therapist to records which need updating (20). Certain third-party payers, such as Medicare, may require a daily entry in the treatment record.

Documentation of progress is not confined to the written record. Also used to depict progress are:

Diagrams (109);
Appropriately designed rubber stamps (101);
Office copying equipment for hand function (76);
Motion pictures (65);
Slides and graphs (27);
Mimeographed forms;
Videotape (70).

Flow sheets are especially beneficial for noting patient response, particularly for items that have numerical value and temporal relationships (35, 104). Flow sheets should have patient identification, date, and a section for immediate comments. Evaluative procedures such as goniometry and muscle testing, and therapeutic procedures such as the tilt table, ultraviolet irradiation, progressive resistive exercise, and walking endurance, are all amenable to flow sheet usage. It is essential that the physical therapist predict the signs and data that he wishes to collect on a flow sheet; this takes forethought and planning (103).

Problem Oriented Record

As early as 1956, Weed began work on what is now known as the Problem Oriented Medical Record (POMR) (104). The premise of the "Weed system" is that form and structure enhance, rather than restrict, the ultimate delivery of health care.

Phillips noted that the POMR is directed toward 1) organizing data around problems, 2) preserving medical logic as well as medical data, and 3) assessing the quality of care given to the patient (88).

There are four elements of the POMR (35, 57, 88, 104, 105): 1) the data base, 2) the problem list, 3) the initial plan, and 4) the progress notes. Weed insists that there must also be continual enumeration, evaluation, integration, and audit of all the patient's problems (104).

The data base consists of the information that is needed to formulate the comprehensive problem list. The initial collection of data should be as complete as possible. The use of trained paramedical personnel as interviewers is encouraged, as is the use of branching computerized medical history questionnaires (104). An important factor is standardization of data input from each patient, so that the physician is in a position to comprehensively identify all problems. All evaluative procedures, such as those commonly carried out in physical therapy, should be a part of the comprehensive data base. Standardization of the information required for the data base cannot be overemphasized (94).

The problem list which evolves from the data base serves as a table of contents and index for the patient's record (29, 51, 104). Milhous notes that each problem should be identified at the level it is understood (77), i.e., as a diagnosis, a physiological finding, a symptom or physical finding, or an abnormal laboratory report. The problem list should include physical, social, medical, psychiatric, demographic, and economic factors (51, 77, 88, 104). Each problem is numbered and assigned an active or inactive status. As new problems appear, they are given a subsequent number and placed on the list. Previous inactive problems should also be placed on the list at the initial workup of the patient.

The third element is the initial plan. This list of plans, both diagnostic and therapeutic, is numbered sequentially according to the problem number in the problem list. The plans may call for 1) collection of further data, 2) treatment with specific procedures, or 3) plans for education of the patient about his illness and his part in managing it (104). The area of patient education is extremely important (77, 82, 104). Weed noted that studies of compliance in medical therapy indicate a level of noncompliance after discharge as high as 25 to 50 percent (104). The plan for patient education must be one which helps the patient to learn best from his own experience, and must provide for ample repetition of basic concepts (104). The specific variables to be followed on the progress note or flow sheet must be identified. The variables thus identified are the most important part of the plan, for they constitute the monitor or feedback system (104).

Chronological and multidisciplinary progress notes, each titled and numbered according to the problem they assess, serve as a mechanism of follow-up on each identified problem (104). Progress notes consist of narrative notes, flow sheets, and a discharge summary. Notes entered by physicians, nurses, and allied health personnel are included in a chronological manner. The acceptable format is subjective data (S), objective data (O), assessment (A), and plan (P) (SOAP) (51, 57, 104). The subjective data (S) include any patient complaint or symptomatic data. The objective data (O) include factual observations, tests, and measurements. The assessment (A) deals directly with the subjective and objective portions of the note, and forms an important part of the feedback mechanism which allows the physician to relate the subjective and objective findings back to the original problem (104). The plan (P) is the immediate plan relating back to the subjective and objective data and the assessment. The final portion of the progress note is the discharge summary. Each numbered problem on the patient's list should have an adequately summarized note when the patient is discharged.

Several physical therapists have published on the topic of POMR as it relates specifically to physical therapy (31, 35, 57). Two of these, Feitelberg (35) and Hill (57), give detailed instructions which allow implementation of POMR in the "working clinic" situation.

The POMR is a means of facilitating improvement in five areas (88): patient care, health education, health care evaluation, clinical research, and computerization. All of these factors are essential to the future of physical therapy. The multidisciplinary notes of the POMR lead to teamwork within the health professions, and intellectual stimulation and incentive for all health workers (88). Anderson (9) and Shaughnessy and Burnett (96) note the distinct advantages of the POMR in long-term care facilities and illness. Weed indicates that the more tightly coupled patient care and education can become by means of the medical record, the greater will be the benefits to all members of the health care team (106). Schell and Campbell refer to the Weed "Multiplier Effect" (94). They note that, with the POMR, every time a health care worker is audited someone is educated; and everytime someone is educated, the patient receives better care. The POMR, then, with its approach to standardization, has built in the necessary "feedback loop" which is essential to meaningful and equitable peer review. What is audited is the professional's ability to collect proper data, identify and assess the problems, and plan procedures to attack the problems. The numbered progress notes leave a trail which can identify the logic the worker uses as (s) he gathers more information, treats the problem, and educates the patient (104).

Finally, as Weed notes (103–107), the POMR provides the basis for computerization of the entire medical record. Standardization is essential for computerization. The POMR will take hospital records a long way toward that goal (51, 88, 104).

Multidisciplinary Progress Notes

Multidisciplinary, chronological progress notes (3, 29, 35, 77, 103), such as those used in the POMR, have the following advantages: total progress is noted quickly by the written record; important observations from all disciplines are available; concise recording is encouraged; the number of different forms in the total record is reduced; the concept of the team approach to patient care is enhanced; and progress notes tend to be recorded more quickly in an attempt to maintain chronological sequence. The obvious disadvantages are (3): the chart cannot be used by more than one person at a time for recording or reviewing; occasional statements may appear to be in conflict between physician and allied health worker, thus creating doubt as to the patient's progress; the progress notes are separated from the more detailed reports of evaluations or therapy in any particular department; and, it is necessary that each note be signed with both the name and discipline of the recorder.

The advantages of multidisciplinary progress notes become more obvious when the POMR is used (104). Multidisciplinary progress notes result in precisely defined building blocks which make the total team effort cumulative toward solution of the particular problem at hand. This sort of thoughtful organization of the medical record can only be advantageous. Anderson notes that standardization will mean development of common approaches to evaluation, establishment of criteria for defining patient problems, chronological recording of pertinent events, objective measurement of evaluations and treatment, and the use of standardized terms (6). This leads to the eventual possibility of electronic data processing in the area of progress notes and patient care records. But it will always be the continual responsibility of the physical therapist to provide the accurate input information.

Discharge Summaries

The final progress note should be in the form of a discharge summary (109). This note should relate specifically to the initial note. If a home program is developed for the patient, a copy of the program must be inserted in the chart. The reason for discharge should be noted, in the event of readmission. Any return appointment given to the patient should also be recorded for reference.

The discharge summary should be a capsule view of the patient's progress during therapy. It should include the reasons for referral, the initial treatment plan, the evolved progress, and the patient's status at the time of discharge. Summary forms, such as those noted by Burger (18) and Garfinkel (42) are acceptable examples. The patient discharge summary is an important report, and considerable care should be spent in developing it. Progressive patient care as discussed by Patierno (83) cannot function effectively, if at all, unless the record or a summary of the record of patient care is readily available to move along with the patient.

Whenever a home program is established for the patient, a copy, identifiable as to patient, physical therapist, and date, should be inserted in the patient's record. The goals of the home program should be made evident to the patient and his family before the day of discharge. The program should be specific to the goal in mind. The program must be tailored to the needs of the individual patient. Routine mimeographed home programs with generalized nonspecific exercises result in nonspecific activity at home. The use of audiovisual techniques, such as suggested by Magill (70), integrates sound teaching and learning techniques into the home instruction process. The written program should include the purpose, methods, frequency, and specific precautions. Equipment or supplies needed for the home program should be indicated to the family prior to discharge, so that the purchase can be made and the equipment installed before the patient arrives at home. Involvement of the family in the home program and the importance of their motivational role should be continually emphasized.

A mechanism for the reinforcement of the home program must be developed. A home visit is preferred, because this gives the therapist an opportunity to observe the patient in his home milieu. Follow-up visitation by a home health physical therapist is ideal, providing there is good interagency communication. Patient re-evaluation in the physical therapy department at specific intervals is also acceptable. In either case, problems concerning the patient's progress or his home program should be reviewed and corrected, and adequate notation made on the patient's record.

The importance of follow-up and follow-through care in health systems will undoubtedly become even greater. Concepts such as the health maintenance organization will necessitate continual and periodic review of patient progress, even during the "healthy state" (86). As Brook et al. indicated, the prevalent disease entities are chronic conditions for which only management, not cure, is possible (15). The increased incidence of chronic conditions demands expanded work for physical therapists in the area of follow-up and follow-through health care.

ADMINISTRATIVE RECORDS

Departmental Data and Statistics

Statistical records in physical therapy deal primarily with frequencies or counts of patients, patient visits, patient treatments, and staff personnel and the interrelationship of these factors, to demonstrate departmental growth. As the progress note is the clinical building block, the statistical record is the administrative building block.

As in all scientific activities, the data collected should relate directly to the intent and purpose of the study (21, 79). Prior to determining the data to be collected, the physical therapist must determine what it is he wishes to reinforce or demonstrate. Data have been collected in physical therapy for the following reasons (114):

1. Departmental planning. Caseloads, staffing patterns, space and equipment needs, and service requirements can be determined by reviewing data collected in the department.
2. Budgetary and cost analysis factors. Justification for existence must be

based on return for investment and that return must be justified by either monetary or service value. Documentation of either of these factors requires objective data.

3. Scheduling. Efficient scheduling in the department can be completed only when a pattern of work flow is identified. This pattern can be identified only by objective data.

4. Standards of work. Performance of various categories of workers is more easily evaluated if accurate measurement of the caseload is documented.

5. Organizational control. Optimum use of personnel, space, and equipment will be possible only when based on objective data.

There is no simple way to outline the types of data and statistics that may be advantageous. Again, the type of data collected must be based on intended use. A distinction should be made between summary data and statistics. Summary data are totals, such as in total number of patient visits per day, per month, or per year. An example of a statistic is the average number of patient visits per month during a given calendar year. An average or mean, like a median—as in the median salary of all chief physical therapists in a geographic area, is a statistic that represents a central tendency of collected data (23, pp. 87–90). Because data are collected on some variable of interest (e.g., patient visits, modalities used, or sources of referrals) over some period of time (e.g., day, month, or year), any expression of summary data or a statistic should include statement of the variable and the period of time. To conserve space, the examples given below present only the variables, and most of these can be thought of as either summary data (cumulative totals) or statistics (averages), or both.

In general, summary data and statistics concerning the following factors and variables have been determined to be of value (4, 6, 21, 114):

1. Information related to patients and treatments:
   a. number of modalities per patient;
   b. number of daily visits per patient;
   c. daily charge, based on modality or time;
   d. length of time for each treatment;
   e. number of home visits; and
   f. travel time for home visits.

2. Information related to staff personnel:
   a. cumulative totals for each staff person on the preceding variables;
   b. number of patients treated;
   c. number of patient visits and number of treatments;
   d. number of inpatients;
   e. number of outpatients;
   f. number of modalities used;
   g. number of new patients; and
   h. number of staff working days.

3. Information related to departmental growth:
   a. cumulative totals and averages on variables in both of the preceding categories;
   b. number of discharges;
   c. condition of patients at time of discharge;
   d. number of discontinuances, and brief reasons for discontinuation;
   e. number of patients per type of treatment;
   f. number of patients per insurance carrier, Medicare, private pay, or welfare;
   g. number of referrals or patients per individual physician;
   h. number of referrals or patients per speciality group;
   i. number of referrals per individual health or welfare agencies; and
   j. number of referrals or patients per geographic region.

Analysis of the purpose for the data will dictate the form for recording and presentation. As with all medical records, this form should be accurate, brief, clear, and understandable. A total system of recording data which begins at the daily level, and progresses through weekly, monthly, and yearly accumulations, will begin to bring order out of chaos. As in reporting the results of scientific studies, methods of organizing data (23, pp. 83–86) and presenting data in graphs and charts (24) will help bring further order to this activity.

Several methods of recording data have been reported or are in use, from handwritten methods (17, 21, 28) to more advanced coding systems which use the standard of time or modality for reporting (7, 44, 55, 65, 110). As standardization continues, the eventual outcome will be the use of a computer input terminal within the physical therapy department for recording the required data (22, 81, 95, 111). In the meantime, the kinds of data collected will be different from Canada to Oklahoma, from the one extreme of combining the patient abstract (80) to the other of combining the patient referral (36) with the patient billing form.

The value of a monthly statistical report, which culminates in an annual report, cannot be overestimated. Such reports are of great value for information and education of administrative personnel, for orientation of new staff members, and for public relations (4, 6, 114). The monthly statistical report should be delivered to administrative personnel on a prompt and regular basis. Such a report should show the total on each variable for the month, the cumulative total on each variable for the year to date, and comparative data from the previous year (114). Again, the variables included will depend on the information you are attempting to convey. At the minimum, the report should contain information on the number of patients treated, the number of new referrals, the number of patient visits, the number of modalities (by individual modality and total), and a review of the department income to date (114). If your hospital is on a computer system, it is up to you to see that these types of summary data are placed in the hands of proper administrative personnel, including yourself. Other variables, as discussed in the foregoing paragraphs, may also be included in the computer printout.

The annual report should be a comprehensive and goal-oriented document describing the entire service operation of the department over the previous year. The annual report should be made available to staff personnel, personnel in the administrative hierarchy, and other interested public and consumer-oriented groups. The annual report should include a synoptic review of the monthly statistical reports. Other factors to be included would be (4, 6, 21, 114):

1. A recapitulation of the stated goals for the department from the previous year;
2. An overall review of the department achievements in light of last year's goals;
3. Personnel changes;
4. Personnel activities: both professional and supportive personnel, and both job related and community activities;
5. Department educational activities;
6. Department research activities;
7. Equipment purchases;
8. Space renovation or changes;
9. Departmental administrative organization;
10. Operational problems during the past year;
11. Goals and objectives for the department for the coming year.

As in all scientific endeavors, the study of departmental data and statistics should raise questions (114). How you learn from the questions raised, and how you benefit from the information collected, will be up to you as an imaginative administrator.

Personnel Records

Records or forms will be needed for employment applications, certification or registration of professional personnel, change of status, evaluation (facility, staff, and student), attendance, vacation and sick leave, leave request, expense records, professional malpractice and liability coverage, and continuing education participation. The topic of evaluation is currently receiving rightful emphasis. There is considerable material available which can serve as a beginning point for the development of records and evaluation forms in personnel management (12, 16, 37, 54, 60, 62, 68, 73, 79, 88, 107, 113). Performance appraisal systems, such as those outlined by Haimann (52) and Longest (69), serve a dual purpose—evaluation for promotion and compensation purposes, and evaluation for employee self-improvement. Because of the importance attached to performance appraisal, much care should be given to determining the proper performance variables to be detailed on the forms.

Financial Records

The records involved in fiscal management of the department include those on income and expenditure, assets and liabilities, cost analysis, and other budgetary matters. Regulations dictate that a list of prices or charges for services rendered within the department be posted and/or be available for consumer information. The cost analysis mentioned earlier should be the basis for these charges (19, 43, 44, 75, 91).

Equipment Records and Other

Appropriate equipment records include procurement and depreciation files for all equipment, and a record of equipment maintenance. The Occupational Safety and Health Act, effective 1971, requires preventive maintenance on all equipment. Good administrative and clinical practice have long dictated the need for preventive maintenance, but this Act demands it. The written maintenance record and check list must be kept in either the physical therapy department or the maintenance department. The record must be kept up to date. Other hospital records and forms, most of which originate from other departments, are work orders, housekeeping requests, central supply requisition forms, supply inventory forms, information release forms, photograph release forms, accident or incident forms, and a myriad of others.

ELECTRONIC DATA PROCESSING

Electronic data processing (EDP) in physical therapy began during the decade of the 1970's (6, 7, 55, 92, 93, 111), and is likely to undergo explosive growth during the decade of the 1980's. The work that has been reported provides a solid base upon which to build. One difficulty, however, is that, in such a rapidly changing field, "here today, gone tomorrow" is the theme song of the computer hardware and software salesman as well as the programmer. At best, we can try to identify some principles and speculate on eventualities.

Every phase of the medical record will benefit from computerization (104). This is particularly true of the comprehensive data base. The difference between computerized records and noncomputerized records lies not only in what has been recorded, but in the ability to know exactly what has not been recorded (49). The computer, properly programmed, can gather baseline data without involving the physician in this time-consuming process (81, 95, 104). A computer cannot perform miracles; it cannot take an irregular and unstructured record and create a logical document (33). The precision must come from the minds of the individuals who determine what constitutes a sound data base. This data base must then be translated into standardized documentation.

Anderson (7) notes that in the initial steps of EDP there must be 1) a definition of the type of treatment activity that takes place in physical therapy, 2) a designed input form, and 3) an acceptable output form if the information is to be used by others. He further notes (6) that the initial requirement of any program involved with EDP is identification of 1) items about which you have information, 2) providers of the information, and 3) transactions that take place in physical therapy. In physical therapy, the items are the patients, the providers of information are the therapists, and the transactions are treatment procedures and their results. Patient identification is via the admitting office information or a suitable numbering system for outpatients, and can be by number, initials, or last name. Transactions which take place in physical therapy are transformed into a numerical code which quantifies evaluation, treatment, and results (6, 93).

Many types of input vehicles are available for computer usage in medical care. These include but are not limited to:

Prepunched cards (55);

Mark Sense (6);

Online teletype (111);

Cathode ray tube with light pencils (88);

Label touch terminals (95);

Cathode ray tube with touch sense (66);

Video matrix terminals (22);

Optical scan (6);

Color bar identification (81).

Data storage units include magnetic drums, discs, tapes, and card decks. Retrieval can be by cathode ray tube, time ordered flow sheet, or high speed printers. Teleprocessing equipment, with online and real time capabilities, allows interaction and dialogue with the computer (22, 81, 95). The rapid advances in this area would make drawings or photos obsolete before this manuscript is published.

The desired characteristics of the terminal for input are ease of operation, accuracy, auditability, and economic feasibility (81). The total online hospital system should have the final capability of building and maintaining the patient's record; maintaining record of census; construction and communication of messages, including orders and financial and statistical information; providing for inquiry into data storage; and providing for addition of system modules (81). In addition, hospital departments should be able to receive orders directly from the nursing station terminal, send messages free format (bypass computer) to the nursing station, and have internal pricing and data gathering capabilities.

Davis talks of a prototype for future computerized medical records (26). He noted that success will depend on the standard file structure, supported by all of the programs within the structure. The key, again, is standardization, structure, and organization. Van Brunt indicates that computers will, if not actually reduce absolute cost of data storage and transfer, at least make larger volumes of data manageable for the same cost (100). He feels that presently available hardware (computer equipment) is probably adequate for most medical applications. Some of the problems that he discusses include 1) the present need for a duplicate system to provide for programming and testing; 2) software (recording material) reliability problems: periodic degradation of the system can be expected; 3) error detection schemes with a greater degree of sophistication and a greater provision for rapid error recovery; and 4) the need for education of medical personnel with regard to the objectives, scope, and rationale of the system.

One problem which has been worked on by Weed (104), Savander and Stutz (93), and others (51) is the development of a "standardized patient's problem index." Anderson (6, 8) indicates that the major reasons that patients need physical therapy can fairly accurately be categorized as patient problems. Thus, the structure for computer language would be available for documentation of activity in the clinic.

Present usage of EDP in physical therapy includes selection and documentation of administrative statistics, billing, patient scheduling, patient transportation scheduling (55, 111), and the recording and retrieval of patient evaluation, treatment, outcome, and demographic information (6, 7, 92, 93).

CONCLUSIONS

A review of the uses, requirements, principles, and forms of physical therapy records will never be complete. New uses and forms appear with developing and changing areas of practice and patterns of delivery of health care services. New requirements and forms appear with new or changing governmental programs. New evaluation forms appear almost monthly in the published literature, and the area of automated records changes as rapidly as the technology that makes those records possible. Only the principles seem to endure.

The entire concept of health care records will continue to undergo change (46). Even as that occurs, physical therapy will continue to expand into practice settings other than traditional locations, and new, or new combinations of, record uses, requirements, and forms will emerge. Different practice settings have different record keeping needs (10, 33, 38, 39, 42, 59, 74, 86, 87, 102). As physical therapy takes the long overdue step into rightful responsibility in preventive health measures, documentation through record keeping will become even more exacting. Evidence to support this contention is available in the field of medicine (89).

Automation of records will certainly increase and become more nearly universal. Automation requires standardization. Standardization improves reliability. Eventually, automation and standardization will make total audit of clinical activities possible, reliable, equitable, and speedy. Then, perhaps, records will best serve their primary purpose: the betterment of patient care.

With this edition I again say to you—the written record is a building block. This chapter constitutes but one rock. BUILD ON IT!

Acknowledgments. The author wishes to acknowledge the assistance of the Harley E. French Medical Library at the University of North Dakota in conducting the literature search with the aid of the Medline-Remote Access Retrieval Service, National Library of Medicine, Bethesda, Maryland. The assistance of several physical therapist colleagues whose personal communications were of much value is also gratefully acknowledged.

References

1. Acheson, E.D.: The patient, his record and society. Med. J. Aust., *2:* 351–355, 1972.
2. Adkins, H.V.: Personal communication. Rancho Los Amigos Center, Downey, California, 1979.
3. American Hospital Association: *Medical Records Departments in Hospitals, Guide to Organization.* American Hospital Association, Chicago, 1972.
4. American Hospital Association: *Physical Therapy Service. A Guide to Organization and Management.* American Hospital Association, Chicago, 1965.
5. American Hospital Association: *Five-Year Index of Physical Therapy, 1971–1975.* American Physical Therapy Association, Washington, 1976.
6. Anderson, L.R.: Electronic data processing physical therapy. Prog. Phys. Ther., *1:* 150–167, 1970.
7. Anderson, L.R.: Physical therapy records. Phys. Ther., *50:* 1187–1197, 1970.
8. Anderson, L.R.: Standardization of the physical therapy record. Phys. Ther., *56:* 911–913, 1976.
9. Anderson, T.P.: Problem orientation of medical records-advantages in long-term illness. Postgrad. Med., *50:* 274–277, 1971.
10. Bartz, A., Offerman, D., Weston, L., Johnson, P., Miller, B., and Hock, D. (unpublished project): *Physical Therapy in the Public School System,* Department of Physical Therapy, University of North Dakota, Grand Forks, 1979.
11. Berni, R. and Readey, H.: *Problem-Oriented Medical Record Implementation,* Ed. 2. Mosby, St. Louis, 1978.
12. Bianco, E.: The medical audit: Powerful tool for upgrading care. Hosp. Prog., *51:* 72–74, 1970.
13. Bonkowsky, M.L.: Adapting the POMR to community child health care. Nurs. Outlook, *20:* 515–518, 1972.
14. Briggs Printing Company: Physical therapy forms. Briggs Printing Company, Des Moines, Iowa.
15. Brook, R.H., Appel, F.A., Avery, C., Orman, M., and Stevenson, R.L.: Effectiveness of inpatient follow-up care. N. Engl. J. Med., *285:* 1509–1514, 1971.
16. Brown, C.R., Jr., and Uhl, H.S.M.: Mandatory Continuing Education—Sense or Nonsense: JAMA, *213:* 1660–1668, 1970.
17. Brown, M.E.: The record folder: Five suggested uses. Phys. Ther. Rev., *32:* 628–633, 1952.
18. Burger, J.L.: Rehabilitation summary form. Phys. Ther., *46:* 1181–1184, 1966.
19. Burton, B., Hewitt, D.R., Patton, F.L., Graves, D.A., Magistro, C.M., and McKillip, J.D.: Guidelines for the establishment of fees for physical therapy services. Phys. Ther., *45:* 730–733, 1965.
20. Caldwell, R.W.: Suspense File: A system for keeping progress reports. Phys. Ther., *49:* 166, 1969.
21. Carlin, E.J.: Principles of record keeping. Phys. Ther. Rev., *37:* 369–373, 1957.
22. Computer receives order from doctor, sends information back to everyone. Mod Hosp., *119:* 68–71, 1972.
23. Currier, D.P.: *Elements of Research in Physical Therapy.* Williams & Wilkins, Baltimore, 1979.
24. Currier, D.P.: How to present data in figures and tables. Phys. Ther., *55:* 768–772, 1975.
25. Daniel, W.W., and Coogler, C.E.: Some quick and easy statistical tests for physical therapists. Phys. Ther., *54:* 135–140, 1974.
26. Davis, L.S.: Prototype for future computer medical records. Comput. Biomed. Res., *3:* 539–554, 1970.
27. Demopoulos, J.T., and Williams, D.: Use of graphs to record patient progress. Phys. Ther., *50:* 670–672, 1970.

28. Dempsey, M.W.: Physical therapy records. Phys. Ther. Rev., *35:* 377–379, 1955.
29. Dinsdale, S.M., Mossman, P.L., Gullickson, G., Jr., and Anderson, T.P.: The problem-oriented medical record in rehabilitation. Arch. Phys. Med. Rehabil., *51:* 488–492, 1970.
30. Dreyfus, E.G., Minson, R., Sbarbaro, J.A., and Cowen, D.L.: Internal chart audits in a neighborhood health program: A problem-oriented approach. Med. Care., *9:* 449–454, 1971.
31. Echternach, J.L.: Use of the problem-oriented clinical note in a physical therapy department. Phys. Ther., *54:* 19–22, 1974.
32. Edsall, F., Darnell, R., Ivanoff, J., and Kobus, K.: Procedure for facilitating physical therapy research. Phys. Ther., *57:* 1138–1142, 1977.
33. Esley, C.E.: Medical records. Hospitals, *46:* 135–140, 1972.
34. Everest and Jennings, Inc.: Wheelchair evaluation and prescription forms. Everest and Jennings, Inc., Los Angeles, California.
35. Feitelberg, S.B.: *The Problem Oriented Record System in Physical Therapy.* University of Vermont, Burlington, 1975.
36. Ferretti, M.J.: Personal communication. St. Anthony Hospital, Oklahoma City, 1973.
37. Fessel, W.J., and Van Brunt, E.E.: Assessing quality of care from the medical record. N. Engl. J. Med., *286:* 134–138, 1972.
38. Field, F.W.: Communication between community nurse and physician. Nurs. Outlook, *19:* 722–725, 1971.
39. Fields, R.D.: Physical abilities of the mentally retarded child. Phys. Ther., *49:* 38–46, 1969.
40. Forkner, C.E.: Delivering the essentials of medical care to all segments of the population. Am. J. Med. Sci., *262:* 194–203, 1971.
41. Ganti, A.R., Piper, N.J., and Nagy, E.J.: Quality control program—An aid to quality care. Phys. Ther., *54:* 233–238, 1974.
42. Garfinkel, M.: Proposed record form. Phys. Ther. Rev., *34:* 238–240, 1954.
43. Gee, D.A., and Hickok, R.J.: Cost analysis development for a physical therapy department. Phys. Ther., *42:* 383–387, 1962.
44. Gee, D.A., and Hickok, R.J.: Developing unit costs for physical therapy modalities. Phys. Ther., *42:* 713–718, 1962.
45. Gee, D.A., and Hickok, R.J.: Differentials in physical therapy procedures by patient category. Phys. Ther., *43:* 721–724, 1963.
46. Gertzog, J.: The changing concept of medical records. Public Health Rep., *85:* 673–679, 1970.
47. Gonella, C.: Designs for clinical research. Phys. Ther., *53:* 1276–1283, 1973.
48. Gordon, B.L.: Terminology and content of the medical record. Comput. Biomed. Res., *3:* 436–444, 1970.
49. Graves, S.: Better records: First step to better quality. Mod. Hosp., *116:* 105–108, 1971.
50. Guilford, J.P., and Fruchter, B.: *Fundamental Statistics in Psychology and Education,* 5th ed., pp. 13–14. McGraw-Hill Book Company, New York, 1973.
51. Gullickson, G.G., Jr.: Personal communication: *Procedure Manual for Problem-Oriented Medical Records* (unpublished). Department of Physical Medicine and Rehabilitation, University of Minnesota Hospitals, Minneapolis, Minnesota, 1973.
52. Haimann, T.: *Supervisory Management for Health Care Institutions,* pp. 195–211. Catholic Hospital Association, St. Louis, 1973.
53. Hammer, N.L.: Opening the department. Phys. Ther., *45:* 1162–1164, 1965.
54. Heap, M.F.: The need for effective selection of personnel in physical therapy departments. Phys. Ther., *49:* 7–14, 1969.
55. Heath, J.C.: Personal communication: *Computerized Workload Reporting System-Physical Therapy* (unpublished). Naval Hospital, Oakland, California, 1972.
56. Health, J.F.: Only patient can permit examination of his record. Mod. Hosp., *117:* 71–73, 1971.
57. Hill, J.R.: *The Problem-Oriented Approach to Physical Therapy Care—Programmed Instruction.* American Physical Therapy Association, Washington, 1977.
58. Holmes, G.: Personal communication. Crippled Children's Hospital and School, Sioux Falls, South Dakota, 1973.
59. Holmes, T.M.: A public health agency solves the problem of written prescriptions. Phys. Ther., *39:* 90–91, 1959.

60. Hoog, J.: Physical therapy standards of practice and audit procedure. Phys. Ther., *51:* 176–181, 1971.

61. Hoog, J.: Professional standards for quality patient care. Phys. Ther., *49:* 1364–1368, 1969.

62. Hulten, A., Kerstall, J., Olssonk R., and Svanborg, A.: A method to calculate nursing load. Scand. J. Rehabil. Med., *1:* 117–125, 1969.

63. Inaba, M., and Jones, S.L.: Medical documentation for third-party payers. Phys. Ther., *57:* 791–794, 1977.

64. Johnson, F.J., ed.: *The Fifty-Year Index of Physical Therapy.* American Physical Therapy Association, Washington, 1971.

65. Koch, K.: Personal communication. Medical Center Rehabilitation Hospital, Grand Forks, North Dakota, 1979.

66. Krismer, J., and Cordes, J.F.: Computer systems: Problem-oriented record begins with the patient. Mod. Hosp., *115:* 81–83, 1970.

67. Lehmukuhl, D.: Techniques for locating, filing and retrieving scientific information. Phys. Ther., *58:* 579–584, 1978.

68. Lister, M.: Performance evaluation of the new staff member. Phys. Ther., *46:* 387–390, 1966.

69. Longest, B.B., Jr.: *Management Practices for the Health Professional,* pp. 126–130. Reston Publishing Company, Inc., Reston, Virginia, 1976.

70. Magill, G.: Self-produced videotapes aid in home instruction. Phys. Ther., *58:* 1092, 1978.

71. Magistro, C.: Personal communication. Pomona Valley Community Hospital, Pomona, California, 1973.

72. Mayo, N.E.: Patient compliance: Practical implications for physical therapists—a review of the literature, Phys. Ther., *58:* 1083–1090, 1978.

73. McDaniel, L.V.: The critical incident method in evaluation. Phys. Ther., *44:* 235–242, 1964.

74. McKee, J.I., and Vaughn, D.T.: The organization and management of a private physical therapy practice. Phys. Ther., *51:* 1100 1106, 1971.

75. McKillip, J.F., and Dicus, R.G.: Cost analysis and cost accounting. Phys. Ther., *51:* 79–80, 1971.

76. Metcalf, V.A., and Yeakel, M.H.: Documentation of hand function with the use of office copying equipment. Phys. Ther., *52:* 935–943, 1972.

77. Milhous, R.L.: The problem-oriented medical record in rehabilitation management and training. Arch. Phys. Med. Rehabil., *49:* 182–185, 1972.

78. Molander, C.O., and Weinmann, B.: A new chart system for recording joint measurements. Phys. Ther. Rev., *21:* 88–90, 1941.

79. Moore, M.L.: A guide for the chief physical therapist: Organizational responsibilities, Phys. Ther. Rev., *33:* 161–165, 1953.

80. Murnaghan, J.H., and White, K.L.: Hospital patient statistics-Problems and prospects. N. Engl. J. Med., *284:* 822–828, 1971.

81. National Cash Register Co.: NCR hospital online communication and data collection system. National Cash Register Co., Dayton, Ohio (1972).

82. Pascasio, A.: Continuing education for quality health care. Phys. Ther., *49:* 257–264, 1969,

83. Patierno, R T · Progressive patient care. The practical answer to rising hospital costs. Phys. Ther., *48:* 234–236, 1968.

84. Patton, F.L.: Justification and general cost of space, Phys. Ther., *45:* 1165–1170, 1965.

85. Patyon, O.D., Seubott, S., DeFlora, G., and Mayer, V.: Quality of patient care and a peer review system: A model. Phys. Ther., *51:* 296–299, 1971.

86. Perry, J.W., and Nechasek, J.E.: Health maintenance: Challenge for the allied health professions, in Institute Proceedings, State University of New York at Buffalo, School of Health Related Professions. Buffalo, New York, 1971.

87. Peyton, R.G.: Personal communication. Sports Medicine Education Institute, Inc., Atlanta, Georgia, 1980.

88. Phillips, D.F.: The problem-oriented system. Hospitals, *46:* 84–88, 1972.

89. Physician's Attitude Survey: Record keeping-A medical obsession. Med. Opinion, *2:* 2: 18–20, 1973.

90. Physician's Record Company: Physical therapy record forms. Physicians' Record Company, Berwyn, Illinois.

91. Price, J.W.: Setting rates for physical therapy services. Phys. Ther., *49:* 265–268, 1969.
92. Savander, G.R.: Development of an outcome assessment and informational system for physical therapy: A multi-institutional project. Phys. Ther., *57:* 891–896, 1977.
93. Savander, G.R., and Stutz, R.N.: Electronic data processing of physical therapy services. Phys. Ther., *53:* 1046–1054, 1973.
94. Schell, P.L., and Campbell, A.T.: POMR-Not just another way to chart. Nurs. Outlook, *20:* 510–514, 1972.
95. Searle Medidata, Inc.: Information 320. Searle Medidata, Inc., Waltham, Massachusetts.
96. Shaughnessy, M.K., and Burnett, C.N.: Implementation of the problem-oriented progress note in a skilled nursing facility. Phys. Ther., *59:* 160–166, 1979.
97. Stokes, J., III.: Is the patient's record more important than the patient: Med. Opinion, *2 (2):* 13–16, 1973.
98. Teca Corporation: Electrodiagnostic record form. Teca Corporation, White Plains, New York.
99. Tufo, H.M., and Speidel, J.J.: Problems with medical records. Med. Care, *9:* 509–517, 1971.
100. Van Brunt, E.E.: The Kaiser-Permanente Medical Information System. Comput. Biomed. Res., *3:* 477–487, 1970.
101. Walters, G.C., and Hoth, M.: Aid for recording gross evaluation. Phys. Ther., *44:* 179, 1964.
102. Watkins, A.L.: Physical therapy in the home-Standing orders and priority listings. Phys. Ther. Rev., *31:* 219–222, 1951.
103. Weed, L.L., Wakefield, J.S., and Yarnall, S.R.: *Implementing the Problem-Oriented Medical Record,* ed. 2. MCSA, Seattle, 1976.
104. Weed, L.L.: *Medical Records, Medical Education, and Patient Care.* Case Western Reserve University Press, Cleveland, 1971.
105. Weed, L.L.: Medical records that guide and teach. N. Engl. J. Med., *278:* 593–600, 1968.
106. Weed, L.L.: Medical records that guide and teach: Concluded. N. Engl. J. Med., *278:* 652–657, 1968.
107. Weed, L.L.: Quality control and the medical record. Arch. Intern. Med., *127:* 101–105, 1971.
108. Wessman, H.C.: Absenteeism, accidents of rehabilitated workers. Rehabil. Rec., *6:* 15–18, 1965.
109. Wessman, H.C.: Progress notes. Phys. Ther., *45:* 727–729, 1965.
110. West, D.M.: A coding system for reporting treatment services. Phys. Ther., *49:* 863–868, 1969.
111. Westrem, D.: Personal communication. North Memorial Hospital, Minneapolis, Minnesota, 1973.
112. Wolf, S.L., and Clifford, H.C.: Interacting with computer personnel in performing clinical rehabilitation research. Phys. Ther., *56:* 178–183, 1976.
113. Wood, M.L.: Appraisal of professional performance. Phys. Ther., *42:* 565–569, 1962.
114. Zimmerman, J.P.: Statistical data. Phys. Ther., *49:* 301–302, 1969.

chapter 5

QUALITY ASSURANCE

James A. Armour and Gary R. Savander

The purpose of this chapter is to provide the physical therapist with the background and principles of a systematic approach for reviewing the quality of the patient care he provides. The external forces that have stimulated quality assurance activities and current quality assurance requirements are discussed to provide a perspective for the quality assurance system we propose throughout much of the chapter. The proposed system brings together for the first time, in an integrated way, the two aspects of quality assurance with which we have had experience, namely, outcome assessment and retrospective audit. We show that these two aspects, which represent, respectively, monitoring the results of care and assessing the results of care, are complementary and that both can be used effectively in improving the results of care.

Fifteen years ago, public discussion of the quality of physical therapy care in America was practically nonexistent. During the 1970s, it became one of the major issues of the profession. The U.S. Government has launched a massive and unprecedented regulatory effort to develop a nationwide system of quality assurance. This effort is known as the Professional Standards Review Organization (PSRO) program. This program encompasses small community hospitals, large teaching hospitals, and regional, state, and federal facilities. If the current quality assurance efforts are expanded to include nonhospital institutional care, ambulatory care, and care reimbursed by private health insurance as well as government programs, annual expenditures for quality assurance in health care may well exceed billions of dollars. While this expansion seems less likely now than when we began to prepare this chapter, because of the economy and action on the federal budget, the growing public and professional interest in quality assurance in health care is intensifying.

As physical therapists, we have an obligation to understand quality assurance and our role in it, and to recognize that objective self-examination is a necessary extension of our service as professionals. A functional quality assurance system can improve the physical therapy manager and practitioner as well as improve physical therapy care.

Clarification of Terms

This chapter uses the term quality assurance to include the objective measurement of the quality of care and a concomitant responsibility to correct deficiencies when they are identified. To measure the quality of care, one may study structure, process, or outcome. The quality assurance system we propose in this chapter places primary emphasis on outcome assessment, with the findings of the assessment serving as a means of identifying problems of process or structure.

We know of no better descriptions of the terms structure, process, and outcome, for the purpose of this chapter, than those found in the American Physical Therapy Association guidelines for developing a system of peer review (1).

Structure

A review of structure is an assessment of organization, staffing and staff qualifications, rules and policies governing professional work, records, equipment, and physical facilities. The assessment may include a judgment of the adequacy as well as the presence of the element of structure being examined.

Process

Process assessment is based on the degree or extent to which the physical therapist conforms to accepted professional practices in providing services. The various approaches to care, their application, efficacy, adequacy, and timeliness are considered. A process review requires that considerable attention be given to developing and specifying the standards to be used in the assessment.

Outcome

Outcome assessment is based on the condition of the patient at the conclusion of care in relation to the goals of treatment.

Assessment of outcomes provides a means for reviewing the practitioner, the services, and events which led to the results of care. The results of outcome assessment ultimately may lead to the evaluation of the basic treatment procedures and modalities of physical therapy and validation of the approaches to patient care. Outcomes are the ultimate manifestations of effectiveness and quality of care.

HISTORICAL PERSPECTIVE

Health professionals have long understood that information based on actual performance is important. The concept of systematic performance evaluation based on health care *results*, however, was slow to gain general acceptance within the health professions.

As early as 1863, Florence Nightingale proposed a system for collecting hospital statistics. She realized that the availability of such information could make it possible to systematically improve hospital treatment. Her efforts to implement a widespread system for collecting data were only partially successful.

Shortly after World War I, Ernest Codman made a major effort to encourage his fellow physicians to analyze the "end results" of their activities in order to determine their strong and weak points and to use this analysis to direct their care of patients. Codman believed that physicians should provide care to *only* those patients for whom they cared well, and that they should avoid providing care to those patients for whose care they were not qualified (4). Codman's efforts to encourage his colleagues to adopt his method of "end result" analysis were unsuccessful. As a result of his noble attempt, however, he is considered the father of the outcome patient care audit systems that gained widespread use in the late 1970s.

Efforts to encourage and develop evaluation of patient care were practically nonexistent for about 50 years, from the time of Codman's work until interest was renewed in the 1960s. This hiatus in development was probably due to a belief that medicine was more art than science and to a reluctance to subject individuals to peer scrutiny.

The early call for end result analysis lost out in favor of a more easily instituted concentration on hospital standardization. This later effort, an important one, was aimed at developing and implementing minimal standards for hospitals in terms of the staffing, organization, and physical facilities necessary for adequate care. The early hospital standards established by the American College of Surgeons provided a foundation for later quality review efforts based upon standardization. The general assumption behind such standardization was that, given qualified health professionals working in the proper setting, good care will result (4).

In 1952, the Joint Commission on Accreditation of Hospitals (JCAH) was established to take over the standard setting function from the American College of Surgeons. The standards established by the JCAH were also directed to minimal achievement of environmental requirements. The assumption underlying the JCAH standards continued to be that if the structure and process required by the standards were met, the professional judgments made in the approved environment would have the best chance of being optimal. This approach continued the concentration on evaluating the hospital, rather than the actions of the health professionals who worked within the hospital.

It is important to note that these hospital standards, determined largely by the opinions of experts and authorities who intended to assure the quality of care, were being developed at the same time that profound social changes were occurring which would affect the whole notion of quality assurance and responsibility for it.

During the period from the mid-1950s into the early 1970s, America entered the "Age of Consumerism." Ralph Nader exposed the automobile industry, the Viet Nam war fostered distrust of authorities and experts, politicians suffered from an eroded image climaxed by presidential disgrace, and the United States military failed to win two wars. The public gradually demanded a more active role in guiding its destiny and protecting its future (7).

It was inevitable that public attention and skepticism relating to expert opinion and authority would also focus in on health care. Aided by ever increasing media coverage of health care events and accomplishments, the public became better informed about the capabilities and the problems of modern medicine and the health care industry.

The assumed responsibility for assuring the quality of care began to shift from the professions to the public sector. In 1965, the courts held that a hospital was responsible for the quality of care rendered by a member of the medical staff. The landmark Darling v. Charleston Community Memorial Hospital case uprooted the time honored charitable immunity that had been granted to hospitals.

The 1965 Medicare legislation set out the conditions of participation for health care providers in federally funded programs. The conditions incorporated many structure and process elements as previously defined. One of the conditions was utilization review, the objective of which was to assure that the level of hospital care was medically necessary and that the quality of care met the expectations of the medical staff. The focus at that time was less on the cost of health care and more on the purchase of health care services that were appropriate, timely, and adequate.

In 1967, government began to realize that the cost of the federally funded health care programs was exceeding earlier estimates. So, stricter utilization review requirements were established that were also applied to the Medicaid program. At this point, many health care professionals began questioning government's intent in the implementation of programs proposed to measure the quality of care: was government measuring the quality of care, as intended in 1965, or attempting to control the cost of care? By the early 1970s, it had become apparent that the revised utilization review requirements were not totally successful in meeting the objective of controlling costs or in measuring the quality of care. The Congress of the United States responded to this state of affairs in 1972 through passage of the Bennett Amendment to Title VI of the Social Security Act (12). This amendment provided for the establishment of Professional Standards Review Organizations (PSROs), which were to review and exercise greater control over the costs and the quality of care for patients covered under federal programs: Medicare, Medicaid, Maternal and Child Health, and Crippled Childrens programs (8). This legislation also provided for the review of nonphysician health care services and for local review, in the sense that health professionals who provide a specific service are to be involved in reviewing that service. The legislation specifically mentioned physical therapy as one example of the nonphysician services that should be involved. The law represented a major shift in the focus of responsibility, in spite of the provision that PSROs use the services of hospitals having the capability of conducting review activities. The vast majority of hospitals, under both Medicare and Medicaid, retained their utilization review and quality-of-care responsibilities, but the ultimate responsibility shifted to an external organization, the PSRO (3).

In 1971, the JCAH revised its hospital standards and directed increased emphasis on quality maintenance activity. Various quality review mechanisms were in use at this time, and many of these mechanisms had been stimulated by the Medicare Law which required medical evaluation. The purpose of medical care evaluation under Medicare, and the focus of many of the quality review mechanisms, was essentially to monitor the use of the hospital and its resources.

These quality review mechanisms suffered additional shortcomings (4). Some mechanisms consisted of a subjective, unsystematic review of small numbers of randomly selected patient charts, in which one physician reviewed one patient chart at a time using his own implicit criteria. At the opposite extreme, others collected, abstracted, and displayed such a great volume and diversity of data that in-depth review was obscured. Many of the review mechanisms were aimed at minimizing the risk of third party retrospective denial of reimbursement, and others were aimed primarily at discovering priorities for continuing medical education. The latter stopped short of demanding analysis of alleged suboptimal practice and of attributing confirmed deficiencies to their sources. Techniques for screening out acceptable records not requiring peer review either did not exist or were ineffective, so the review process was too time-consuming for those least able to afford the time—the practitioners. Validity and reliability were suspect in almost all the quality review mechanisms, and not until recently was there any systematic programmed action to correct problems unless the problems were so gross that the need for correction was readily apparent (4).

Taken together, these shortcomings in the quality review mechanisms prompted the development of the Performance Evaluation Procedure (PEP) by the JCAH. The PEP provided a structured mechanisms by which the effects of actual performance could be assessed. Designed primarily to assess care provided by the physician, the PEP required modification to meet the needs of physical therapists who wished to use the method. Such a modification was made by one of us (9).

Early in the 1970s, the Board of Directors of the American Physical Therapy Association (APTA) adopted standards for physical therapy services and standards for the physical therapy practitioner. These standards were subsequently updated, adopted by the APTA's House of Delegates in 1975, and last revised in 1980 (2). The APTA has defined these standards as, "The profession's statement of conditions and performances which are essential for quality physical therapy service and patient care." "Adherence to these standards," the APTA states, "will assure the provision of an acceptable level of patient care."

The early development of the APTA's standards documents created a basis for the establishment of guidelines for developing a system of peer review, adopted by the House of Delegates in 1975 (1). The system of peer review addressed in these guidelines is voluntary, educative, and nonpunitive and includes assessment of structure, process, and outcome.

While APTA was developing its standards and peer review documents, some individual physical therapists were actively developing methods of patient care assessment (9–11).

REQUIREMENTS

The two major forces that are influencing quality assurance development in the United States today are the Joint Commission on Accreditation of Hospitals (JCAH), a voluntary but quasipublic accrediting agency, and the federally mandated Professional Standards Review Organizations (PSROs). Health care professionals who practice in hospitals and those who practice in institutions that provide services to federal beneficiaries find themselves in a reactive position attempting to comply with the standards established by these agencies. The reluctance of the health professionals to objectively evaluate the quality of services they provide coupled with an informed public and the spiraling cost of health care appears to be the major reasons for this state of affairs.

JCAH Requirements

In April 1979, the JCAH revised its quality assurance standard for hospital accreditation. This revision stimulated feverish activity by hospitals to understand the new quality assurance standard and to assure compliance with it. The standard states (5):

> There shall be evidence of a well-defined, organized program designed to enhance patient care through the ongoing objective assessment of important aspects of patient care and the correction of identified problems.

The "well-defined, organized program" addresses the hospital as a whole. This part of the standard requires a written, fully integrated quality assurance program that ultimately reports quality assurance results to the Board of Trustees of the hospital. An example of a hospital wide quality assurance program, reflecting a plan for information reporting, is shown in Figure 5.1 (6). The physical therapy quality assurance program must be an integral part of this whole program.

The physical therapy reviews must be fitted into the overall hospital wide quality assurance program and provisions made to report the findings to the Board of Trustees when appropriate. The JCAH dropped its requirements

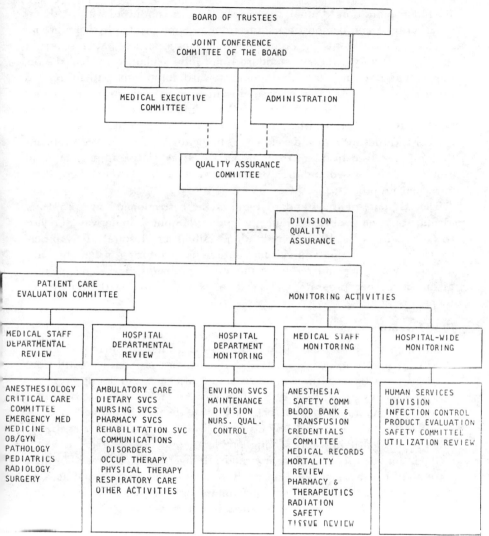

Figure 5.1.   Quality assurance program organizational structure chart (6).

that a certain number of reviews (medical audits) be done annually *per hospital*, but this does not affect the frequency of physical therapy service reviews. Standard I of the section on Rehabilitation Services/Programs in the JCHA Accreditation Manual requires a quarterly review of physical therapy services (5).

The phrase "on-going objective assessment" in the JCAH quality assurance standard requires predetermined criteria for all monitoring and assessment activities in the quality assurance process. In physical therapy, as specified under Standard I of the section on Rehabilitation Services/Programs in the

JCHA Accreditation Manual, the reviews must be conducted with predetermined criteria and demonstrate input from an appropriate physician group.

The use of the words "assessment of important aspects of patient care" in the JCAH quality assurance standard is not fully explained by JCAH. The implication is clearly one that points toward important patient related problems and activities that have significant potential to improve the quality of patient care. The determination of what is important is a joint decision to be made by involved health care practitioners. The implication for physical therapists is that they must develop ways to identify patient related problems that are perceived by them to be important. The relative importance will most likely be assessed and discussed at the time of the JCAH survey of any particular hospital.

The last part of the standard requires the correction of any problems identified by the quality assurance program. Planning is underway to revise this Standard in the 1983 Accreditation Manual for Hospitals. It is anticipated that this revision will call for continuous monitoring of Patient Care and for identifying and resolving important problems. The departmental quality assurance program will need to be intergrated with the overall hospital program.

PSRO Requirements

Although the JCAH currently appears to exert more influence than the PSROs on quality assurance, the PSROs did demonstrate a growing influence in recent years. The continued growth of this influence is in doubt, however, because the very existence of PSROs is subject to the funding decisions of a congress and an administration bent on cutting the federal budget.

In the last few years, the PSROs began to focus their quality assurance reviews on identifying and solving problems, and on using a variety of methods for identifying, analyzing, and solving these problems. The new wave of PSRO reviews relies on analysis of accurate and up-to-date data bases. The previous health practitioner apathy or resistance in some cases has begun to turn to active support for these activities.

The Social Security Act, as amended in 1972, requires that physicians and hospitals that choose to participate in the Medicare or Medicaid program comply with three obligations:

1. To order or furnish only care that is medically necessary.
2. To furnish care that meets professionally recognized standards of quality.
3. To provide such documentation of the medical necessity and quality of care provided as the PSRO may reasonably require.

The PSRO requirements for medical care evaluation (MCE) are in a state of change. The change appears to be in line with the quality assurance requirements of JCAH, except that the hospitals participating in Medicare and Medicaid are required to conduct a minimum number of MCEs each year.

The Health Care Financing Administration (HCFA) acting on reports submitted by PSROs may invoke sanctions against physicians and hospitals that give Medicare and Medicaid patients excessive or poor quality care. The regulations specifying the procedures to be used for invoking these sanctions, published in the February 20, 1980, *Federal Register*, authorize HCFA to exclude physicians and hospitals permanently or temporarily from participation in Medicare and Medicaid or to assess a fine of up to $5,000 in addition to restitution of any improperly paid claims.

With this enforcement mechanism in place, it should be anticipated the utilization review and medical care evaluation programs of hospitals will be reviewed with closer scrutiny by PSROs, hospitals found wanting will be placed on provisional status or sanctions may be recommended if appropriate.

The major thrust of the PSROs continues to be toward review of care provided by physicians, but many PSROs are initiating review of care provided by nonphysicians, as was called for in the 1972 legislation. As PSROs continue to upgrade their data collection and summarizing capabilities, they will be in a better position to identify a wider range of programs in the quality of health care. As they increase their attention to nonphysician services, data concerning physical therapy services will most likely be collected. If problems with the physical therapy service are identified, the physical therapy service will be expected to address the problems. Review of the problem areas with PSRO-approved criteria will be expected, and the physical therapy system for quality assurance must be prepared to meet this expected sequence of events.

Trends in Requirements

While physical therapists should familiarize themselves with the quality assurance requirements promulgated by the JCAH, and by regulation for the PSRO program, we cannot emphasize enough that the details of the requirements change periodically but the principles and objectives are becoming more clear, uniform, and durable. Quality assurance in physical therapy will be best served by development of a system that meets these principles and objectives. Such a system, which will meet the needs of the physical therapy service as well as the requirements of external agencies, is proposed in the remaining sections of this chapter.

QUALITY ASSURANCE SYSTEM

Avedis Donabedian has been quoted as stating, "An efficient system for monitoring care should have least two components: one that sifts large numbers of cases and identifies those most likely to contain defects of management and a second that subjects questionable cases to detailed and definite professional evaluation (4). One can elaborate upon Donabedian's remark but not improve it. He "says it all" in one sentence.

A system for quality assurance should have the capability to monitor, assess, and improve the patient care results obtained by the department. The physical therapy department's quality assurance system should be developed and implemented with the following objectives: evaluate the level of patient care results for the department; evaluate the level of patient care results of each physical therapist; relate patient care results to specific diagnostic groups, therapeutic activities, and intensity of services; relate level of patient care results to productivity information; improve documentation; and assist in management's decision-making process.

The quality assurance system we describe and propose in the remainder of this chapter is designed to follow Donabedian's sage advice and to achieve the objectives set out above. The system is based upon our experiences.

As presented here, the quality assurance system focuses on monitoring the results of care, assessing the results of care, and improving the results of care.

MONITORING THE RESULTS OF CARE

When a department embarks on a quality assurance system the first task is to decide those items of information which will enable the department to monitor the results of its activities and the factors that may influence those results. While this monitoring could be an end in itself, in our proposed quality assurance system the step of monitoring is a means for sifting large numbers of cases and identifying those most likely to contain deficiencies in patient care. Monitoring, then, is a necessary step prior to assessing the results of care in order to identify problems that should be corrected to improve the results of care.

One of the first decisions to be made is that of including in the data collection either the total patient population or a sample of the patient population seen in the physical therapy department. We suggest that the most desirable system is one that includes all patients and has the capability of identifying and retrieving data on specific groups of patients.

The items in the data base should include those that are consistent across all types of patients and that will yield data that can be realistically and meaningfully summarized. Adhering to these principles in a results-oriented quality assurance system raises the next decision to be made—that of documenting patient care outcomes in a way that can be applied to all types of patients and that can be realistically and meaningfully summarized. One of us has devised just such a method that can be used to monitor the results of care. The method defines outcomes in terms of the achievement of goals of each patient's treatment (10, 11).

The goals of treatment are operationally defined to include the full range of patient variables important in physical therapy (e.g., strength, range of motion, coordination, etc.), and to permit the rating of achievement of the goals in a uniform manner. A list of example goals, selected and further developed from a more complete list of goals devised by one of us for electronic data processing and a multi-institutional project (10, 11), is shown in Figure 2.

A. Increase Strength
   Show an increase in strength that allows involved body parts to perform functional activities.
B. Increase Range of Motion
   Show an increase in range of motion that llows involved body parts to perform functional activities.
C. Prevent Contractures
   Show that no decrease or loss of joint range of motion occurs throughout all four extremities.
D. Increase Coordination
   Show an increase in coordination that allows patient to perform functional activities.
E. Increase Endurance
   Show an increase in endurance that allows patient to perform functional activities.
F. Decrease Pain
   Show a decrease in pain, allowing patient to perform functional activities.
G. Decrease Spasticity
   Show a decrease in spasticity, allowing patient to perform functional activities.
H. Decrease Abnormal Sensory Feedback
   Show a decrease in abnormal sensory feedback, allowing patient to perform functional abilities.
I. Improve Balance
   Show an improvement in balance that allows the patient to perform functional activities.
J. Independent Transfer Activities
   Show that patient performs all transfer activities independently.
K. Independent Ambulation
   Show that patient ambulates independently, with or without assistive devices and on level surfaces, for distances that are functional for him or her.
L. Decrease Gait Deviations
   Show a decrease in gait deviations, allowing patient to ambulate functionally.
M. Independent Elevation Activities
   Show that patient ascends and descends stairs and curbs independently, with or without assistive devices.
N. Independent Other Functional Activities
   Show that patient performs all other functional activities independently.
O. Learn Home Program
   Show that patient understands and performs correctly a specific home program directed toward his or her functional needs.

Figure 5.2.   Selected list of goals for use in monitoring results of care.

A three-category scale is used for rating the achievement of these goals: Yes (Y) means *Goal Achieved*, Partial (P) means *Progress but Goal Not Achieved*, and No (N) means *No Progress towards Goal*. This method of rating the achievement of goals does not rule out the need to perform and record more precise measurements used in evaluating patients. Measurements of muscle strength or force, joint range of motion, activities of daily living performance, and so forth, still serve their usual purposes in this system, and in addition provide the basis for selecting each patient's goals.

A distinct advantage of the goal list and the three-category rating scale described above (see Fig. 5.2) is one of placing all important patient outcome variables on the same results-oriented scale of measurement. This approach permits summarizing both the absolute numbers and the percentages of goals achieved, partially achieved, and not achieved, either in particular groups of patients or in all patients. For example, this summarizing capability can be applied to groups of patients according to diagnosis, age, sex, referring physician, responsible physical therapist, or type of therapeutic activity within a particular diagnostic group. This same summarizing capability can be applied to the department as a whole; and, if several departments adopt the same goal list and rating scale, summaries can be made both within and across these departments (10).

For the purpose of the quality assurance system we propose in this chapter, a primary advantage of the method described above is that it provides an efficient means of sifting large numbers of cases in order to identify those in which deficiencies of care are more likely to have occurred. An example of this sifting and screening is provided later.

Other Uniform Data

Treatment outcomes or the achievement of selected goals may vary as the result of several contributing factors over and above what is done to or with patients in a treatment program. We believe that the data base for monitoring the results of care should include data on these contributing factors, as well as on the elements of the physical therapy program and the achievement of goals.

Figure 5.3 presents an example patient data sheet that can be used in a facility that has electronic data processing capabilities (10). The reader should study this Figure and notice the kinds of variables on which relevant data might be collected, as well as the fact that some of the information to be recorded on the sheet would have to be coded for input to the computer. Figure 5.4 shows an example of a simplified form that could be used to collect relevant data in a facility that does not have electronic data processing capabilities. A computer is helpful but not necessary for monitoring the results of care in our proposed system. The chief advantage of having computer capability lies in being able to collect and process much more data, in much less time than can ever be done by hand, and this can affect both the reliability and the validity of monitoring the results of care.

Summary Reports on All Patients

The methods described above can be used to obtain summary reports for comparisons over time, for comparison of an individual physical therapist with the department, or for comparison of the department with other departments in similar settings. Tables 5.1 and 5.2 show examples of the kinds of summary reports that can be generated for these purposes (11). The

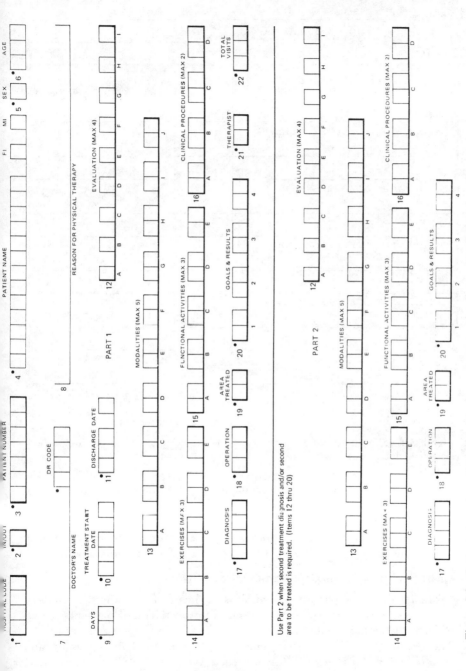

Figure 5.3. Patient data sheet for use with electronic data processing. (Reprinted with permission from G.R. Savander. Phys. Ther., *57*: 893, 1977.)

PATIENT INITIALS_____   PATIENT IDENTIFICATION NO._____

DIAGNOSIS_____   AGE_____

TREATING THERAPIST NO._____

	Achieved	Progress But Not Achieved	Not Achieved
GOAL:			
CLINICAL PROCEDURES USED:			
GOAL:			
CLINICAL PROCEDURES USED:			
GOAL:			
CLINICAL PROCEDURES USED:			
GOAL:			
CLINICAL PROCEDURES USED:			
GOAL:			
CLINICAL PROCEDURES USED:			

TOTAL NUMBER OF PATIENT VISITS:_____

Figure 5.4. Simplified patient data sheet for monitoring results of care without electronic data processing.

greater the quantity of data to be summarized, the more helpful it will be to have access to computer capabilities.

These summary reports are useful in monitoring and assessing the results of care on all patients, but our proposed system needs yet to describe how to use the data on goal achievement to select charts for the audit process.

Chart Selection for In-Depth Study

The retrospective patient care audit is the heart of assessing the results of care. This process requires examination, retrospectively, of particular cases. Because of the large volume, not all cases can be examined retrospectively. The implication, then, is that some defensible method for screening and selecting charts for in-depth study is needed. We propose such a method here, using the data on goal achievement described above.

Table 5.1
Summary Report on Individual Physical Therapist[a]

The Mercer Hospital
Analysis of Physical Therapy Service by Therapist
as of 10/31/72

Report 6830-M

	Therapist 02				
	65 and over	2			
	Under 65	9			
	Male	3			
	Female	8			
	Total Patients		11		
Code 0	Diathermy	34			
1	Ultra sound	90			
2	Microwave				
3	Infra-red	5			
4	Electrical stimulation	8			
5	Ultra violet				
6	Rythmic constrictor	4			
7	Cervical traction				
8	Intermittent compression				
9	Medco-sonlator				
	Total Modalities		141		
1	Deep				
2	Superficial				
	Total Massage				
1	Chronaxie				
2	Manual Muscle Test				
3	Postural Evaluation				
	Total Evaluation				
0	Passive Range of Motion	120			
1	Active Assistive	122			
2	Active	74			
3	Resistive	33			
4	Forced (stretching)				
5	Crutch walking				
6	Gait Training	1			
7	Pre prothetic				
8	Prosthetic				
0	Other				
	Total Exercise		350		
1	Whirlpool	2			
2	Hydrocollator (hot packs)	93			
3	Paraffin bath				
4	Hydromassage				
5	Ice massage				
	Total Hydrotherapy		95		
	Total Treatments			586	3.1	Average treatments per visit
	Goals Yes	16		76.1%	Achievement
	No	2		9.5%	Nonachievement
	Partial	3		14.2%	Partial achievement
	Visits	184		16.7	Average number of visits

[a] Reprinted with permission from G. R. Savander and R. N. Stutz. Phys. Ther., *53:* 1052, 1973.

Table 5.2
Summary Report on Department[a]

		The Mercer Hospital Analysis of Physical Therapy Services as of 10/31/72				

Report 6820-M

	Department Total					
	65 and over	6				
	Under 65	29				
	Male	12				
	Female	23				
	Total Patients		35			
Code 0	Diathermy	46				
1	Ultra sound	160				
2	Microwave					
3	Infra-red	9				
4	Electrical stimulation	13				
5	Ultra violet	1				
6	Rythmic constrictor	3				
7	Cervical traction	32				
8	Intermittent compression	29				
9	Medco-sonlator	19				
	Total Modalities		312			
1	Deep					
2	Superficial					
	Total Massage		9			
1	Chronaxie					
2	Manual muscle test					
3	Postural evaluation					
	Total Evaluation					
0	Passive range of motion	120				
1	Active assistive	136				
2	Active	83				
3	Resistive	40				
4	Forced (stretching)					
5	Crutch walking					
6	Gait training	4				
7	Pre Prosthetic					
8	Prosthetic					
9	Other					
	Total Exercise		383			
1	Whirlpool	54				
2	Hydrocollator (hot packs)	181				
3	Paraffin bath					
4	Hydromassage					
5	Ice massage					
	Total Hydrotherapy		235			
	Total Treatments			939	2.5	Average treatments per visit
	Goals Yes	42			65.6%	Achievement
	No	8			12.5%	Nonachievement
	Partial	14			21.8%	Partial achievement
	Visits	367			10.4	Average number of visits

[a] Reprinted with permission from G. R. Savander and R. N. Stutz. Phys. Ther., *53:* 1052, 1973.

To illustrate the method, suppose that we have chosen to study patients who have had a cerebrovascular accident (CVA) and that this decision was made after monitoring the achievement of goals. If you will look again at Table 5.2, note that 65.6 percent of the goals were achieved by the physical therapy service. Suppose that a similar printout specifically for patients with a diagnosis of CVA revealed that only 40 percent of the goals were achieved, that is, almost 26 percent below the departmental average. This discrepancy may indicate a problem and would justify further study.

A list of patients with a diagnosis of CVA could easily be generated from the data base maintained by the computer system (note that diagnosis was one variable recorded in Fig. 5.3). Such a list might look like the abbreviated example in Figure 5.5, in which is recorded the patient name (initials), patient number, number of visits, and goal results. This same list could be generated manually by summarizing the kind of information that would be obtained by using the simplified patient data sheet shown in Figure 5.4.

To select charts on cases in which deficiencies of care *may* have occurred,

Patient	Patient No.	Number of Visits	Goal Results
S.J.	18090621	30	P/A P/B Y/K Y/J Y/M Y/O DC'd to home
P.M.	18137745	15	Y/A Y/C Y/K Y/I DC'd to boarding house
U.A.	18124420	27	P/K P/A Y/C Y/E DC'd to nursing home
U.N.	18129270	18	P/A Y/C P/G Y/K Y/J N/M
K.P.	18132480	17	P/A P/K Y/E Y/I Y/C DC'd to home
C.T.	18114363	20	Y/C P/A P/K Y/E Y/J P/M DC'd to rehabilitation center
D.M.	18122879	16	Y/A Y/C P/K P/M Y/I N/J DC'd to home

Key: Numerator of each ratio refers to rating goal achievement. Y = Yes; P = Partial; N = No. Denominator of each ratio refers to specific goal (see Fig. 5.2). DC'd = Discharged.

Clarity of *Goal Results*

Patient	Goal Results
S.J.	P/A P/B Y/J Y/K Y/M Y/O
P.M.	Y/A Y/C Y/I Y/K
V.A.	P/A Y/C Y/E P/K
V.N.	Y/A Y/C P/G Y/J Y/K N/M
K.P.	P/A Y/C Y/E Y/I P/K
C.T.	P/A Y/C Y/E Y/J P/K P/M
D.M.	Y/A Y/C Y/I N/J P/K P/M

Figure 5.5. Example goal achievement summary on individual CVA patients.

the suggested criteria for selection are:

1. All charts with one or more goals rated N (e.g., patients V.N. and D.M. in Figure 5.5; *and,*
2. All other charts in which 50 percent or more of the goals are rated P (e.g., patients V.A. and C.T. in Figure 5.5).

Note that the charts of patients S.J., P.M., and K.P. in Figure 5.5, would not be selected for retrospective audit.

We believe that this method of chart selection for audit is *efficient*, in the sense of providing a means for sifting through large numbers of cases, and *effective*, in the sense of identifying those cases most likely to reveal deficiencies of care that can be corrected. In addition, the elements of this method make possible the future study of the reliability and validity of chart selection, and they circumvent the shortcomings of other quality review mechanisms discussed earlier (see Historical Perspective).

Other Monitoring Methods

It is possible to establish other monitoring methods that are less comprehensive than the goal-achievement patient data collection system described above. To monitor, by definition, is to watch, check, or keep track of for a special purpose. Monitoring is a process in which criteria or standards are used to review actual practice in order to identify those areas requiring in-depth study, or to determine the results of corrective action. We should monitor an area if it appears to be a problem or if there is significant potential for improving patient care. As an example, we may decide that periodic monitoring of physical therapy discharge summaries would reveal potential problem areas in the care of patients receiving physical therapy. A simple form for this monitor is shown in Figure 5.6.

After monitoring discharge summaries for a period of time, suppose the data revealed that 40 percent of the charts do not have discharge summaries.

Monitoring of Discharge Summaries		
Department: Physical Therapy		
Responsible Person: Director of Physical Therapy		
Frequency of Review: Weekly		
Number of charts: 10		
Criteria:	Yes	No
1. Discharge summary present in chart	——	——
2. The discharge summary compares the initial physical therapy evaluation of the patient with the final physical therapy evaluation of the patient	——	——
3. The disposition of the patient following discharge is stated	——	——

Figure 5.6.   Simple form for monitoring discharge summaries.

At this point, a potential area for improving patient care has been identified. If it is generally accepted that preparing a discharge summary is part of providing quality patient care, corrective action can be taken immediately without further study. The director of physical therapy can inform the physical therapy staff that a discharge summary will be written on all patients receiving physical therapy. The monitor should then be continued to determine if the problem is corrected. Or suppose that the director's discussion with the staff reveals that the physical therapists are dictating the discharge summaries, using appropriate departmental procedures, but that the summaries are not appearing on the closed charts reviewed in the monitor. In this case, the problem may be administrative and the director should pursue it further with the clerical staff and perhaps with the medical records department. If the monitor reveals that the therapists are not comparing the initial evaluation with a final evaluation (criterion 2 in Fig. 5.6), an in-depth review via a chart audit may be indicated. In this case, it will be valuable to compare the achievement of desired patient outcomes, using audit criteria, in the charts failing to meet criterion 2, as identified through the monitor, and in an equal number of randomly selected charts which meet criterion 2.

A similar monitor could be established to check treatment plans written in the patient record.

There are a number of potential elements that could be monitored in the physical therapy department using data sources that are readily available. The keys to successful monitoring are regular performance and annual reappraisal (or more frequent if indicated) to determine the value of the monitor. Ask the question, "Has the monitor identified problems related to patient care or areas with the potential to increase the quality of patient care?" If yes, then the monitor has been valuable and should be continued. If no, then other elements should be monitored instead. In the long run, identification of appropriate monitoring elements will be the key to success of a quality assurance system.

ASSESSING THE RESULTS OF CARE

Once the questionable charts have been identified through the goal achievement monitoring system, assessing the results of care through the retrospective patient care audit can proceed. If a simpler monitoring method is used, the area of concern becomes the audit topic. The audit topic is an area with significant potential for improving the quality of patient care, or a problem area, identified through monitoring.

The audit topic can be a disease (CVA), an operative procedure (below knee amputation), a special evaluation (manual muscle testing), or a problem (inability to walk). Although any topic can be selected, it should be relevant to the patient population being served, and it should have significant potential to improve the quality of care provided.

The method of retrospective review or audit discussed here is the Simplified Physical Therapy Audit, by Saitz, Hoy, and Armour (9). The discussion is intended to help the reader understand the concept and principles of retrospective audit and to appreciate the role of audit in a quality assurance system. The reader who wants to learn the process of audit should consult the original, more extensive source (9) and should attend one or more of the workshops on audit provided for physical therapists.

The physical therapy audit attempts to determine the quality of patient care through review of the patient record. The audit provides an orderly, structured method of comparing actual practice as revealed by the patient record to the expected level of quality of care.

We recommend that the audit or assessment be conducted by a committee, although the format can be used by an individual provided the criteria are objective and the analysis is without bias. The committee must include at least one physical therapist who thoroughly understands the audit process.

Since most audits are retrospective, appropriate records of discharge diagnoses or operative procedures can be obtained from hospital summaries. The study should include records from at least a six-month period to represent a diverse sample. If the time period is too long, say, more than two years, the information in the sample may be contaminated by therapeutic or institutional changes.

The actual number of records reviewed will depend upon the monitoring system used, the topic selected, the hospital size, and available personnel. In the CVA example used in the previous section, the charts were identified through the monitoring process. If a monitor other than the goal-oriented method is used that does not identify specific charts or groups of charts, then 20 records is a manageable number for physical therapy departments of medium-sized hospitals.

The audit includes four distinct steps: 1) development of screening criteria, 2) data retrieved, 3) data display, and 4) data analysis. Before the first step is undertaken, however, the objectives of the audit—the reasons why it is to be conducted—must be defined and agreed to by the committee. The previous monitor can provide much of the information needed to define the objectives of the audit. Discussion of the monitoring information allows the committee to decide which objectives are most appropriate. Once the objectives are defined, it is easier to develop and apply appropriate screening criteria.

Development of Screening Criteria

Developing the screening criteria is not only the most important part of the audit, but also the most difficult. Decisions made at this point carry through and influence the entire study. The criteria should be designed to screen out records most likely representing acceptable patient care from direct physical therapist review. Only those records that do not satisfy one or more screening criteria should be reviewed by the therapists. If a record fails a screening criterion, it does not necessarily imply poor care but means only that the record will be returned for review. Variations from screening criteria can represent acceptable patient care, but this decision must be made by the physical therapists.

Clinically relevant and reliable screening criteria are difficult to develop. Frequently it is possible to evaluate them only after actual use in an audit study. However, the following guidelines will be helpful when developing screening criteria for the first time.

Consider these questions for each criterion:

1. Specifically *what* are you looking for?
2. Do you know *why* you are looking for it?
3. Does it really *make a difference* in patient care?
4. Can it be *measured* in the existing medical record?
5. Can two or more persons, particularly medical data analysts, read the criterion and come to the *same interpretation* of it?

See Figure 5.7 for screening criteria developed for records of patients who have been diagnosed as having CVA. Figure 5.8 presents screening criteria for records of patients who have been diagnosed as having low back problems not attributable to displaced intervertebral discs.

Examination of Figures 5.7 and 5.8 shows that the screening criteria have four components: "elements" (operational definitions of what to look for); "expected ALL or NONE" (a check of whether all or none of the records should show the elements); "exceptions" (exceptions to the all-or-none check on elements); and "explanations for the medical data analyst." The criteria components provide a two-stage sorting mechanism for the medical data analyst to use during record review (Elements and Exceptions) and also directions for summarizing the study (Expected ALL or NONE).

The elements of the screening criteria usually fit into one or another of the categories shown below, and in general one or more elements are developed for each category:

Evaluation (initial or ongoing);
Physical therapy procedure;
Discharge status;
Complications;
Other indicators.

Data Retrieval

The audit procedure reduces the number of records requiring complete physical therapist review either by pinpointing the variations within each record or by assessing the entire record as satisfactory and therefore not requiring therapist review. The medical data analyst performs the time-consuming tasks of obtaining records for the study and then abstracting and summarizing the information from these records. Because the abstracting is

AUDIT FACE SHEET _____   Committee: Physical Therapy Audit Committee   Date: February 1975

Topic Includes: Cerebral vascular accident resulting   Index Codes: ICDA-8   430 -438   _____ Original
                  in hemiplegia   X   Repeat of _____

Excludes: Mortality patients

Patient Population: All patients

Number of records to be reviewed: All, up to a maximum of 20

Number of records available for same period: _____

Time Period __7/74__ to __2/75__

This completed form is an educational resource of the
Pennsylvania Physical Therapy Association Audit Committee

Figure 5.7. Screening criteria for the cerebrovascular accident (CVA) patient. (Reprinted with permission from the Pennsylvania Physical Therapy Association, Inc.)

No.	Topic Elements(s)	Committee Expected All	None	Exception(s)	Date / Explanations for Medical Data Analyst
1	Initial range of motion exam completed	X		None	Initial = before treatment Range of motion (ROM) includes one or more of the following: a. active b. passive c. subluxations
2	Initial motor evaluation completed	X		None	Initial – before treatment Motor evaluation includes one or more of the following: a. muscle strength b. muscle tone c. spasticity d. rigidity e. flaccidity
3	Presence or absence of neurological signs pertinent to physical therapy are re-corded	X		None	Pertinent neurological signs include one or more of the following: a. sensation (pin prick, light touch, deep pressure, tracts intact, tactile descrimination, position sense, stereognosis, proprioception, depth perception) b. coordination (finger to nose, dexterity, balance sitting, standing, kneeling) c. reflexes (increased deep biceps, triceps, knee, ankle, superficial clonus, Babinski) d. cranial nerve disorders (hemianopsia) e. other (dysarthria, Nohman's sigh)
4	Independent ambulation on the level with or without devices	X		Discharge with con-tinued physical therapy treatment	Devices – braces, crutches, cane, walkeret Check physical therapy discharge note or physician's discharge note for Exception Continued physical therapy treatment = a. extended care facility PT program b. nursing home PT program c. visiting nurse for PT

Figure 5.7.—*continued*
SCREENING CRITERIA

No.	Elements(s)	Expected All	Expected None	Exception(s)	Explanations for Medical Data Analyst
4	Continued				d. rehabilitation center e. home health PT program f. continued PT outpatient hospital care
5	Independent ambulation on steps with devices or railing	X		Discharge with continued physical therapy treatment or Unable to ambulate on steps prior to CVA	Check physical therapy notes or physician's discharge notes for Exception Continued physical therapy treatment: a. extended care facility PT program b. nursing home PT program c. visiting nurse for PT d. rehabilitation center e. home health PT program f. continued PT out-patient hospital care
6	Independent in transfer techniques	X		Discharged with continued physical therapy treatment	Check physical therapy notes or physician's discharge notes. Continued physical therapy treatment: a. extended care facility PT program b. nursing home PT program c. visiting nurse for PT d. rehabilitation center e. home health PT program f. continued PT out-patient hospital care
7	Maintain range of motion in the involved upper extremity within normal limits (WNL)	X		Patient reports a sufficient amount of pain to interfere with exercises	Pain factor must be documented in physical therapy notes. WNL is as documented in initial evaluation
8	Maintain range of motion in the involved lower extremity within normal limits (WNL)	X		Patient reports a sufficient amount of pain to interfere with exercises	Pain factor must be documented in physical therapy notes. WNL is documented in initial evaluation
9	Discharge program given	X		None	Discharge program must be documented in the PT notes or as a separate report to a nursing home, an extended care facility, visiting nurse, rehabilitation center home health agency, patient

AUDIT FACE SHEET

Committee: Physical Therapy Audit Committee   Date: September 1975

Topic Includes: Lumbosacral strains and sprains   Index Codes: ICDA-8   846
                Low back pain   728.7
                Lumbago   717.0

                                                         _____ Original
                                                           X   Repeat of Nov. 1974
                                                                       ‾‾‾‾‾‾‾‾‾

Excludes: Displacement of intervertebral discs   ICDA-8   725.1
          (Lumbar and lumbosacral)

Patient Population: 18 - 65 years old

Number of records to be reviewed: 20 per facility
                                  ‾‾‾‾‾‾‾‾‾‾‾‾‾‾‾‾‾

Number of records available for same period: _____

Time Period 1/75 to 8/75
           ‾‾‾‾‾‾   ‾‾‾‾‾‾

          This is an educational resource of the Pennsylvania Physical Therapy
          Association through a grant from the Western Pennsylvania Regional
          Medical Program

Figure 5.8. Screening criteria for patients with lumbosacral strains and sprains, low back pain, and lumbago. (Reprinted with permission from The Pennsylvania Physical Therapy Association, Inc.)

Figure 5.8.—*continued*

SCREENING CRITERIA

Topic Lumbosacral disorders   Committee   Date

No.	Elements(s)	Expected All	Expected None	Exception(s)	Explanations for Medical Data Analyst
1	Initial evaluation completed	X		None	Initial evaluation includes two or more of the following: a. straight leg raising (SLR) b. pain c. muscle spasm d. strength e. sensation f. posture (sitting, standing, walking) g. tenderness h. range of motion (ROM)
2	Reduction of pain and/or tenderness as defined by initial evaluation	X		Physician's intervention with no resumption of PT	Physician's intervention = any of following: a. surgery b. casting c. continous bed rest d. continous traction e. intravenous (IV) treatment f. myelogram
3	Discharge evaluation completed	X		None	Discharge evaluation must be completed within 5 days of discharge and includes two or more of the following: a. straight leg raising (SLR) b. pain c. muscle spasm d. strength e. sensation f. posture (sitting, standing, walking) g. tenderness h. range of motion (ROM)
4	Discharge instructions provided	X		None	
5	Complications Increase in patients's pain and/or tenderness as defined by initial evaluation		X	Notify physician	Physician notification may be verbal or written but must be documented in PT notes

Topic Lumbosacral disorders (continued)

| | | Expected | | Committee | | |
No.	Elements(s)	All	None	Exception(s)	Date	Explanations for Medical Data Analyst
						MDA to record and report to Committee:
						a. Number of charts with a final diagnosis of 300.1 (hysterical component) or 305.1 (pyschogenic origin) listed in physician's discharge summary
						b. Number of visits per patient
						c. Type of treatment given to each patient

completed according to the components developed by the physical therapists and specified on the Screening Criteria form, it does not require clinical judgment. This adds an element of objectivity since a noninvolved person actually reviews the record.

The data analyst codes the results of reviewing each record on special forms. The codes indicate whether the record satisfied the element, the exception, or neither (a variation) for each screening criterion. Data retrieval forms are used to total the results for all records and provide a subtotal for each physical therapist. This information is the basis for the next phase of the audit, the data display.

Data Display

The data display summarizes the medical data analyst's review of all records. It includes the total number of records reviewed, the age and sex distribution of the patients, and the distribution of records for each physical therapist. Specific information collected from the records is arranged into meaningful categories by:

1. Listing the total number of records and the percentage rate satisfying each criterion;
2. Listing individual chart numbers of records not satisfying each criterion;
3. Identifying the physical therapists for these records;
4. Pointing out additional information, including the correlation of multiple criteria for the same record.

Data Analysis

The physical therapists must review the data display and the records that did not satisfy the screening criteria in order to determine the quality of care. This review may indicate that the care was acceptable or that there were deficiencies. When deficiencies are identified, their cause must be determined. Deficiencies may be related to care or to the criteria and method of the audit. If related to care, appropriate actions can involve procedural changes, continuing education, or other corrective actions. If related to the criteria and methods, appropriate changes should be made. The physical therapists' judgments and recommendations concerning the study are then sent to other professional and administrative staff members responsible for the care given by the institution.

Look again at Figure 5.5, the goal achievement summary on individual CVA patients. Recall that we made a decision to study those charts where no progress was made toward one or more goals selected for the patient and therapist to achieve, and those charts where 50 percent or more of the goals were only partially achieved. In our example, the charts to be studied were those of patients U.A., U.N., C.T., and D.M. The number of charts was kept small for illustration, but in actual practice the number of charts on CVA patients in the study would be much larger. You can see that the seven charts listed in Figure 5.5 were reduced to four by the criteria used.

The four charts were perceived to contain potential problems because the achievement of goals was less than acceptable to the physical therapists involved. The four charts (U.A., U.N., C.T., and D.M.) were then compared to the screening criteria in Figure 5.7. These criteria were approved by the physical therapists involved in the study and represented their expression of acceptable care. The medical data analyst (or a trained secretary) then developed a data display that revealed how each of the four charts compared to the screening criteria. Chart U.A. did not meet screening criterion element 4 (independent ambulation) in Figure 5.7, but did meet the exception to the criterion. Chart C.T. did not meet screening criteria elements 4 and 5 (independent ambulation and elevation) in Figure 5.7, but did meet the exceptions to these criteria. Charts U.A. and C.T., as a result of meeting the appropriate exceptions, met the departmental definition of acceptable care.

Chart U.N. failed to meet criterion 5 in Figure 5.7, both the element and the exception. Chart D.M. failed to meet criteria 4, 5, and 6 in Figure 5.7, both elements and exceptions. Because charts U.N. and D.M. failed certain screening criteria, the quality assurance committee was required to review these charts. Suppose that the review of these two charts revealed that the patients were treated by the same therapist, that they had the same physician, that social service had not been consulted, that the disposition of the patients was not documented in the physical therapy progress notes, and that the physical therapy documentation did not include a discharge summary. The physician's progress notes recorded that both patients had been discharged to home.

The quality assurance committee may conclude that the care was deficient in both cases. The problem may be identified as a lack of discharge planning by both the physician and the physical therapist. We discuss possible corrective action for this problem in the next section.

The monitoring process can also be used to identify a problem area for study by random selection of charts rather than by specific chart identification, as in the illustration just described. Suppose the monitor of goals achieved with patients presenting with "low back pain" demonstrated that the department was achieving only 30 percent of the goals. The quality assurance committee could decide to pull a random sample of 20 charts to study this apparent problem. They would develop screening criteria for use by the medical data analyst or secretary for screen these 20 "low back pain" charts. An example of the criteria used in reviewing the charts of patients with low back pain is shown in Figure 5.8. The committee would then review the charts that failed to pass the screening criteria. The actual study in which these criteria were used revealed that the therapists were not adequately evaluating the patients who presented with "low back pain."

IMPROVING THE RESULTS OF CARE

We have discussed the first and second stages of the quality assurance system—monitoring and assessing the important aspects of patient care. The third and final stage is improving the care provided. The monitoring process enables focusing limited resources on problem areas or areas that have significant potential to improve the quality of patient care. The assessment process enables the in-depth study of these areas to determine the nature of the problem and what corrective action can best be applied to fix it. Then, of course, the corrective action must be implemented. If this final step is not completed, the previous work is futile, for it is only through appropriate, corrective change that the quality of care can be improved. To have a quality *assurance* system, it is inherent that the care is not only studied, but also corrected when found to be deficient.

In the CVA example used in this chapter, the quality assurance committee had identified a deficiency involving a lack of discharge planning. The quality assurance committee recommended that the director of physical therapy assure that each patient have a written physical therapy plan of care that includes posthospital plans for the patient. They also recommended that the director of physical therapy discuss the deficiency of care with the involved therapist. A further recommendation was for the quality assurance committee to monitor the CVA patient care by auditing 20 charts in 6 months using criteria 4, 5, 6, and 9 of Figure 5.7.

Fortunately, the hospital in which this study was done had an integrated quality assurance program similar to that in Figure 5.1. The Physical Therapy Quality Assurance Committee reported their findings to the Patient Care Evaluation Committee, and the physician deficiency was addressed by the appropriate medical staff committee.

The low back audit example mentioned in the previous section revealed that the therapists were not evaluating the patients sent to the department for care. In fact, discussion of this at a staff meeting revealed a total lack of continuity with regard to the process of evaluating the patient with low back pain. As a result, one of the senior staff was sent to a continuing education course on evaluation and treatment of the "low back" patient. The senior staff member worked with the Physical Therapy Quality Assurance Committee to establish a protocol for low back evaluation. The protocol was discussed at a physical therapy staff meeting and accepted by the majority of the staff. Six months after the acceptance of the protocol, the charts of low back patients were studied again using the screening criteria in Figure 5.8. Significant improvement was found. The patient sample (20 charts) showed 100 percent compliance with the criterion of a physical therapy evaluation, and satisfaction of criterion 2 in Figure 5.8—the patient outcome criterion—had increased from 40 to 60 percent.

The following list summarizes briefly some additional problems that were actually identified through retrospective audit and the corrective actions that were taken (the list is by no means all inclusive):

1. Failure to document adequately and need to further improve discharge summaries. Monthly staff meetings to discuss documentation were scheduled. Note writing guidelines were developed and adopted (see Fig. 5.9).
2. Need to improve evaluation skills and to develop evaluation guidelines. Six staff members attended 64 hours of class on evaluation and treatment. Evaluation guidelines were incorporated in note writing guidelines (Fig. 5.9).
3. Inability of other health workers to readily find physical therapy progress notes in the open chart. Distinct section for physical therapy notes was added to the open chart.
4. Rehabilitation treatment and evaluation records were not included in the closed chart. Procedure for including these records in the closed chart was adopted.

The examples offered in this section on improving the results of care illustrate the important principle that *THE QUALITY ASSURANCE SYSTEM PROPOSED IN THIS CHAPTER CAN ALSO SERVE TO ASSESS THE EFFECTIVENESS OF CORRECTIVE ACTIONS TAKEN TO IMPROVE THE RESULTS OF CARE.* The methods of monitoring and assessing the results of care, described earlier, can be applied to see if corrective actions actually affect outcomes in terms of goals achieved and screening criteria satisfied.

CONCLUDING REMARKS

Individual, often subjective impressions of why a particular patient or patient type improves, stays the same, or gets worse in the course of receiving physical therapy may still be useful in practice but is becoming increasingly unacceptable as a method of measuring the quality of care. The quality assurance system described and proposed in this chapter is a systematic, objective, and universally applicable method of measuring the quality of care.

The quality assurance system we propose emphasizes the outcomes or results of care, and provides a means of getting at the problems or deficiencies that contribute to poor quality of care. The system is compatible with other segments of the health care industry, and enables one to express the results of measuring the quality of care in a manner that can be understood by persons outside the profession.

One advantage of our proposed quality assurance system that has not been mentioned is that its use will enable any physical therapy service to document and communicate the results of patient care over time. In other words, use of the system will make the service or department better able to describe its principal product.

A. Initial Note (all patients)
1. Mode of transportation to department (optional)
2. Referral diagnosis
3. Other diagnosis or condition that would alter treatments or affect progress
4. Patient's physical status
   a. Range of motion evaluation
   b. Motor evaluation
   c. Neurological evaluation (optional)
   d. Pertinent findings related to diagnosis (optional)
5. Patient's functional status
   a. Transfers
   b. Ambulation
      -level
      -stairs
6. Patient's mental status (optional)
   a. Orientation of patient to time, place, and person
   b. Inability to follow commands
   c. Poor judgement
   d. Language barriers
   e. Attitude or cooperation
7. Goals set
   a. Short term
   b. Long term
8. Treatment plan

B. Progress Notes (as needed per following:)
1. Goal changes
2. Treatment changes
3. Changes in the patient's status and attitude as related to the initial evaluation or prior to progress note
4. Appliances prescribed and dates ordered and delivered
5. Discontinued program
6. If no changes occur a note should be written periodically to document the fact that no change took place. Periodically is best determined by each institution. Acute hospitals need to write more frequently than long term (e.g. 2-3 days as compared to a week).

EVALUATION GUIDELINES
Range of Motion
-active
-passive
-subluxations
   Motor
-muscle strength
-muscle tone
   spasticity
   rigidity
   flaccidity
   Neurological
   (optional)
-sensation
   pin prick, light touch, deep pressure, tactile discrimination, position sense, stereognosis (astereognosis), depth perception
-coordination
   finger to nose, dexterity, balance (sitting, standing, kneeling)
-reflexes
   increased deep (biceps, triceps, knee, ankle), superficial (clonus, Babinski)
-other
   cranial nerve disorders (hemianopsia), dysarthria, Hohman's sign
   Pertinent Findings
-pain
-swelling
-edema
-redness
-skin conditions
   clammy, cold, lesions, petechia

C. Final or discharge note (all patients)
1. Physical evaluation reporting on items documented in the initial note as change or status quo.
   a. R.O.M. evaluation
   b. Motor evaluation
   c. Neurological evaluation (optional)
   d. Pertinent findings related to diagnosis (optional)
2. Patient's Functional status
   a. Transfers
   b. Ambulation
      -level
      -stairs
3. Patient's mental status as compared to initial evaluation or prior progress note.
4. Discharge program outlined and documented as to who received where appropriate.
5. Disposition
6. Number of visits

An educational resource of the Pennsylvania Physical Therapy Association Audit Committ

Figure 5.9. Note writing guidelines for use in physical therapy. (Reprinted with permission of The Pennsylvania Physical Therapy Association, Inc.)

Now, a final word on evaluating a quality assurance system. The evaluation must address two questions:

1. Has the system improved the quality of patient care?
2. Has the system reduced the cost of patient care?

In our current economic environment, these two questions are the "two sides of the same coin"—they are inseparable.

References

1. American Physical Therapy Association: Guidelines for developing a system of peer review, 1975. In *APTA Policy Log*, p. 88–94. American Physical Therapy Association, Washington, 1978.
2. American Physical Therapy Association: Standards for physical therapy services and physical therapy practitioners. Phys. Ther., *60:* 1456–1462, 1980.
3. Goran, N.J., Roberts, J.S., and Rodak, J.: Regulating the quality of hospital care—An analysis of the issues pertinent to national health insurance. In *Quality Assurance in Health Care*, R.N. Ehdahl and P.M. Gertman, eds. Aspen Systems Corporation, Germantown, Md., 1976.
4. Jacobs, C.M., Christoffel, T.H., and Dixon, N.: *Measuring the Quality of Patient Care—The Rationale for Outcome Audit*. Ballinger Publishing Company, Cambridge, Mass., 1976.
5. Joint Commission on Accreditation of Hospitals: *Accreditation Manual for Hospitals*, 1981 Edition. Joint Commission on Accreditation of Hospitals, Chicago, 1981.
6. Mercy Hospital: *Quality Assurance Plan*. Mercy Hospital, Pittsburgh, 1980.
7. Platt, K.A.: Inpatient quality assurance from the viewpoint of the private physician. In *Quality Assurance in Health Care*, R.N. Ehdahl and P.M. Gertman, eds. Aspen Systems Corporation, Germantown, Md., 1976.
8. Sadin, R.R.: Professional standards review organizations—Another quality assurance program. Phys. Ther., *55:* 1315–1319, 1975.
9. Saitz, E.W., Hoy, L.Y., and Armour, J.A.: *Simplified Physical Therapy Audit*. Western Pennsylvania Regional Medical Program, Pittsburgh, 1976 (reprinted in *Patient Care Audit Manual*, American Physical Therapy Association, Washington, 1980).
10. Savander, G.R.: Development of an outcome assessment and informational system for physical therapy—A multi-institutional project. Phys. Ther., *57:* 891–896, 1977.
11. Savander, G.R., and Stutz, R.N.: Electronic data processing of physical therapy services. Phys. Ther., *53:* 1046–1054, 1973.
12. Wright, B.W.: Health care planning—Acts, agencies, and activities of the federal government. Phys. Ther., *60:* 1017–1021, 1980.

chapter 6

PHYSICAL THERAPY AND THE LAW

Donald J. Horsh

This chapter explains the medicolegal principles that are inherent in the practice of the health professions and, more specifically, how these and certain other legal principles apply to the practice of the physical therapy profession. This chapter also updates and discusses the governmental requirements established by legislation that are pertinent to the practice of physical therapy.

The term "medicolegal" is generally used to refer to malpractice and negligence. Malpractice and negligence, although subject to modification by legislation, have their roots in the common law, and the principles of law pertaining to them exist without specific statutory authority. Governmental requirements, on the other hand, are legislative or statutory in nature and are generally concerned with specific programs.

To maintain the distinction between these two broad areas of the law, the chapter is presented in two sections: "Medicolegal Aspects of Physical Therapy" and "Governmental Requirements." While some overlap in the two areas it is unavoidable, the separation into two sections should help clarify the material presented in this chapter and make it more useful to the reader.

MEDICOLEGAL ASPECTS OF PHYSICAL THERAPY

This section discusses the principles and situations that have significant medicolegal implications for the practicing physical therapist; the legal relationships between a physical therapy educational program (school), its students, and the clinical training site; and the elements of contractual obligations.

Shortly after the publication of the first edition of this book in 1974, the cost of malpractice insurance was substantially increased by the major insurance carriers. This increase in cost, along with concern for rising health care costs, created what has been referred to as the "malpractice crisis." This crisis resulted in legislative efforts by several states to help alleviate the situation. The crisis precipitated several changes in the law of the various states—the purpose being to minimize the increasing cost.

The majority of litigation involving malpractice and negligence over the last several years has been directed at physicians, surgeons, anesthesiologists and hospitals. Litigated cases in which physical therapists have been directly involved are very few, and this can probably be attributed to the environment in which the physical therapist practices. For example, the type of patient being treated in physical therapy has completed to a large extent the acute phase of illness or injury; this reduces the risk factor to a great extent and allows more time for planning and implementing a course of treatment. As a further example, the physical therapist to a large degree practices the profession as an employee of a health care organization. How and why this aids the physical therapist will be explained later.

In order to examine the relationship between medicolegal implications and the type of environment in which the profession is practiced, it is necessary to identify the major kinds of arrangements under which the physical therapist provides services:

1. As an employee of a hospital, rehabilitation facility, school system, home health agency, extended care facility, health maintenance organization, group practice, or professional corporation;

2. On a contract basis with one or more of the kinds of organizations enumerated above, that is, as a contractor often representing a physical therapy group practice or professional corporation that may itself employ other physical therapists;

3. As an individual therapist or as a member of a group of therapists providing treatment on a fee-for-service basis.

Undoubtedly other arrangements do exist, but for the purpose of this section the situations enumerated above are sufficient. The basic principles of liability which follow are sufficiently broad to cover other situations.

Liability

A fundamental principle of law is that legal situations arise primarily from contractual relationships or from circumstances that constitute tortious conduct. This principle applies to individuals in the practice of their profession. An exception to this principle is conduct which constitutes a crime. Because criminal law has little implication for the practice of physical therapy, it will not be a subject of this section. Both tort and contract law will be discussed. The major emphasis will be on negligence and malpractice, which constitute the greatest potential for medicolegal difficulty faced by physical therapists in the practice of the profession.

Tortious Conduct

A tort is defined as "a private or civil wrong or injury—a wrong independent of contract—the commission of or omission of an act by one without right, whereby another receives some injury, directly or indirectly in person, property, or reputation" (37). Embraced within the field of tort law are such areas as trespass, assault, battery, false imprisonment, defamatory matter (libel and slander), the right of privacy, negligence, and, where the learned professionals are involved, malpractice.

The physical therapist will not ordinarily be concerned with all of the above named areas that constitute tortious conduct. Several of these areas do, however, merit brief comment. For example, treatment of a patient without his or her consent has been construed to constitute a battery (9). Detaining a patient under circumstances which cause the individual to believe that by leaving the institution serious repercussions will occur has been held to constitute false imprisonment (13). The taking and publishing of pictures and material concerning a patient's condition without valid consent has been construed to be an invasion of the right of privacy (3).

Although the foregoing types of tortious conduct are of concern, they do not pose a major threat to the practicing physical therapist. The major source of concern lies in two other areas of tortious conduct: negligence and malpractice. The primary thrust of this chapter will be directed toward these potential sources of liability.

Negligence

Negligence has been defined "as the failure to do what a reasonable and prudent person would ordinarily have done under the same or similar circumstances of the situation, or doing what such a person under the existing circumstances would not have done and the essence of the fault may lie in omission or commission" (37, pp. 746–747). Negligence is based on the principle that members of society in the conduct of their affairs have a duty to exercise reasonable care so that their activities will not harm the person or property of another. The failure to exercise reasonable care and the situation in which such failure causes injury to the person or property of another to whom a duty is owed give rise to potential liability. In order to sustain an action for negligence, the person claiming injury (the plaintiff) must prove three things:

1. There was a duty owed to the plaintiff by the defendant;
2. There was a breach of that duty under conditions which constituted negligence and the negligence was the proximate cause of the breach;
3. There was damage to the plaintiff's person or property.

Negligence therefore applies to society as a whole. In a case which is considered a landmark, the Court stated:

"the proposition is this. Everyone owes to the world at large the duty of refraining from those acts that may unreasonably threaten the safety of others. Such an act occurs. Not only is he wronged to whom harm might reasonably be expected to result, but he also who is in fact injured, even if he be outside what would generally be thought the danger zone. There needs to be a duty due to the one complaining but this is not a duty to a particular individual because as to him harm might be expected. Harm to someone being the natural result of the act, not only that one alone, but all those in fact injured may complain" (30).

It therefore follows that liability for negligence is applied not only to the original act which threatens the safety of others but also to the logical results which can reasonably be attributed to flow from that original act. It also follows that each and every member of society is legally responsible for his or her own negligent conduct. The physical therapist is therefore personally responsible for any acts which can be construed to constitute negligence and which injure or cause damage to the complaining party or others who may reasonably claim injury as a result of the initial act.

Malpractice

Another type of tortious conduct which has applicability to the physical therapist is malpractice. Although based upon the same basic legal principles that constitute negligence, malpractice has other connotations in that it applies to those areas of activity which have professional significance. Members of a profession, by virtue of special training and licensure (if required), profess and hold out to society that they possess special skills and training. Malpractice is the failure to exercise the training and skills which would normally be exercised by other members of the profession with similar skills and training. More specifically, malpractice has been defined as "the failure to meet the standards demanded and if as a result the patient or client suffers injury the profession (the physical therapist) may be required to respond in damages. Failure to meet the required standards may be due:
1. To the negligence of the practitioner;
2. To his or her ignorance;
3. To willful departure from acceptable practice;
4. To breach of positive law, as by treating the patient without consent" (34, p. 36).

Although malpractice and negligence have some degree of technical difference, as the foregoing indicates, courts and legal authorities have a tendency to consider the actions as being somewhat synonymous. For this reason, the remaining portions of this section will do likewise.

Imputation of Negligence and Malpractice

As indicated earlier, each and every member of society is legally responsible for those acts which through negligence cause injury to others and to whom a duty is owed. A duty to exercise reasonable care, however, is not owed to everyone. The circumstances surrounding the relationships of the parties determine whether or not a duty is owed. For example, it has been held that a trespasser who suffers injury because of the dangerous conditions of the premises is without remedy. Once a trespasser has been discovered, however, and if the defendant negligently injures him, recovery will be allowed (18). The measure of the duty, therefore, rests on the circumstances of the case. Under certain circumstances, negligence may be imputed to a party other than or in addition to the actor who caused the injury or damage.

If a physical therapist owes a duty to another and negligently breaches that duty, a third party may well be required to respond for the injuries sustained by the plaintiff. The circumstances that constitute the arrangement under which the physical therapist practices may implement the doctrine of *Respondeat Superior*.

Respondeat Superior

Respondeat Superior means literally "let the superior respond." The doctrine of Respondeat Superior is based on the principle that the master or employer who accepts the benefits of the servant or the service of the employee must also answer the servant's or employee's liabilities. This principle results in a siutation whereby the employer is held legally liable for the negligent acts of its employee and it is so held even though the employer did not condone or participate in the employee's negligence (31, S. 68). To hold an employer liable under the doctrine, the act complained of must have occurred within the scope of employment, and an employer-employee relationship must have existed (31, S. 70). An act to be construed as being within the "scope of employment" must be one which can reasonably be associated with the position's activities (31, S. 71). The basic test of whether an employer-employee relationship exists is the right of the employer to control the activities of the employee.

The doctrine of Respondeat Superior does not relieve the employee from liability. Every individual is liable for his or her own negligent conduct. The injured party may therefore sue the employee directly for his or her wrongful act. In actual practice, the complaining party will in all probability initiate legal action against both the employer and the employee as defendants in the controversy. From the plaintiff's point of view, this is a rather practical approach, because it is generally assumed that the employer is in a better position financially to satisfy a judgment for damages.

The introductory part of this section identified the three major arrangements under which physical therapists provide services. The first arrangement was one in which the physical therapist provides services as an employee. Ten years ago James stated, "Most insured physical therapists are employees in a hospital, a nursing home, or employees of another physical therapist; thus, a great deal of protection is derived from the doctrine of *Respondeat Superior*" (19). This is most certainly still true. Although the physical therapist is liable for his or her own negligent acts, complaining parties generally initiate legal action against the organization rendering the service, and the employer in most instances carries insurance to protect the organization against such contingencies.

Imputation of negligence can occur under circumstances other than those discussed here and to which another doctrine applies.

Res Ipsa Loquitur

As stated previously, the burden is on the plaintiff to prove the negligent conduct of the defendant(s). To this rule an exception has been pronounced which is legally known as the doctrine of *Res Ipsa Loquitur*, "the thing speaks for itself." The doctrine was first ennuciated in a case tried in England in

1863. The evidence introduced by the plaintiff indicated that he was walking in a public street past the defendant's shop when a barrel of flour from the window above the shop fell and seriously injured him. The plaintiff was unable to actually prove negligence on the part of the defendant since there was no method of proving or showing what caused the barrel to fall. The court reasoned that although the plaintiff could not prove negligence, he should not be without recourse. The court therefore set forth basically the following criteria and further held that, if these criteria are met, a presumption of negligence will be raised against the defendant which the defendant, to avoid liability, must overcome. In order to invoke the doctrine of Res Ipsa Loquitur, the plaintiff must show that the following three conditions exist:

1. What happened does not ordinarily occur without negligent conduct;
2. The instrumentality which caused the injury was wholly in control of the defendant;
3. There was no opportunity for contributory negligence on the part of the plaintiff (7).

The doctrine of Res Ipsa Loquitur has found its way into the health field where it has been used in malpractice cases involving physicians and in negligence cases involving hospitals. A patient was injured in a hospital when the leg on a bed collapsed, causing him to fall to the floor with resulting injuries. A hospital employee was in the process of moving the patient's bed and the patient was in a helpless condition. The court held that the necessary elements to support the doctrine were present (22). The doctrine of Res Ipsa Loquitur could be applied to the activities of the physical therapist. The area which may have the most potential for applying the doctrine is in the use of equipment that is negligently operated or defective, with resultant harm, and where the opportunity for contributory negligence on the part of the patient is not present.

The doctrine of Res Ipsa Loquitur is of particular value to the plaintiff. Normally, the individual claiming injury must prove that it was the defendant's negligence or malpractice which caused the alleged harmful result. Also normally, expert testimony by professional peers is necessary in order to prove malpractice. If, however, the plaintiff can bring the case within the doctrine of Res Ipsa Loquitur, the defendant must prove affirmatively a lack of negligence or malpractice. Quite frequently the defendant is unable to do this, and as a result, the plaintiff often is able to prevail without introducing a single expert witness on his or her behalf. The reluctance of profesionals to testify against their colleagues makes the doctrine a valuable legal method available to the plaintiff for proving malpractice.

Principles of Liability

Practice as Independent Contractor

As previously discussed, each member of society is responsible for his or her own tortious conduct that causes harm to others, but this negligence may be imputed to the employer when the physical therapist is an employee. What is the legal status of the physical therapist who contracts with a health care agency to supply services and the physical therapist who operates his or her own facility and treats patients on a fee-for-service basis? The author's opinion is that the therapists who practice under these arrangements probably occupy the status of independent contractors. This opinion, however, is open to question.

Historically, the physician has been considered an independent contractor when treating patients in a hospital, and the hospital has not been liable under the doctrine of Respondeat Superior for damages sustained by patients as a result of surgical or medical treatment ordered and carried out by the physician. The reason the physician is construed to be an independent contractor is that he is employed by the patient and his or her activities are not subject to control by the administrative officers or employees of the hospital (38). This rule continues to have general application, although exceptions have been recognized in recent years. The most outstanding exception to the rule occurred in a case decided by the Illinois Supreme Court in 1965. In this case (the Darling Case), the patient's leg became gangrenous because a cast was too tight and the physician failed to take proper action. The court held the hospital primarily responsible because certain procedures were lacking, which if implemented should have prevented the result (8). The Darling case could have applicability to the therapist who practices on a contractual basis and, as a result, implicates the health care agency involved. The doctrine has gained considerable acceptance, and health care organizations today are being joined as defendants for many if not all harmful acts which occur on the premises.

Another doctrine that may have some applicability here is that of the *Borrowed Servant*, which has been used in the case of nurses, interns, and residents. This doctrine, based on the doctrine of Respondeat Superior, has been applied to the physician, who so directs the activities of others that he is presumed to control their acts. The physician in this circumstance can be required to answer for the acts of the others even though their salaries may be paid by another party. Although it is conceivable that a physician could so direct the activities of a physical therapist who practices on a contractual basis that it would be possible to invoke the doctrine, the author has been unable to locate any cases in which this occurred. In addition, the applicability of the doctrine in other areas appears to be declining.

The author's contention is that the physical therapist who provides services not as an employee but on a contractural basis or on a fee-for-service basis is probably an independent contractor if the services are performed under conditions which tend to disassociate his or her activities from a hospital or other health care organization. These conditions may place the therapist's activities outside the doctrine of Respondeat Superior, requiring that the physical therapist answer directly for harmful results.

Liability for Acts of Nonprofessional Personnel

The professional physical therapist practicing in a hospital generally is not liable for the negligent acts of nonprofessional personnel under his or her supervision unless he knew or should have known that the individual was not capable of performing adequately the delegated duties. In this instance, the professional and the nonprofessional are both employees of the hospital, and the doctrine of Respondeat Superior may be applied to both.

The above is not applicable to the physical therapist who practices as an independent contractor. In this instance, the therapist is the employer and must respond for harm caused by nonprofessional personnel in the same manner as the hospital or health organization that employs a physical therapist.

The unrelenting rule that every individual is liable for his or her own harmful acts applies to everyone and nonprofessional personnel are no exception. They too must answer for their own acts which constitute negligence.

Contributory Negligence

Although liability is imposed upon defendants for their negligent conduct, it does not follow that this conduct will in all instances result in liability. Liability cases in which both parties (plaintiff and defendant) are guilty of negligence are not uncommon. At common law, contributory negligence is an absolute defense to an action to recover for injuries which have been negligently inflicted (34, p. 182).

In the field of health care, failure by the patient to follow reasonable instructions has been held to constitute contributory negligence. It has also been held that a professional is not liable for a patient's injury that is due to the patient's failure to return for treatment (14).

The results obtained in health care quite frequently depend on how well the patient follows the necessary directions or instructions. It is also not unusual for patients to ignore instructions and suffer harmful effects. When legal action is threatened by the patient, an affirmative defense to such an action could be that the patient's failure to follow instructions constituted contributory negligence. Because negligence on the part of the defendant must be proven by the plaintiff in order to impose liability, the party complaining must generally be free of conduct which can be construed as contributory negligence.

Comparative Negligence

Dissatisfaction with the absolute defense of contributory negligence has been increasing for many years. This dissatisfaction has led to a number of attempts to find some substitute method of dealing with cases in which there is negligence on the part of both parties (31, p. 433). For example, when both parties are negligent, one party may be more negligent than the other. Or, the situation may be one in which the degree of negligence is equal but the amount of damage suffered by one party is greater than that incurred by the other.

In an effort to bring about more equitable decisions on the apportionment of damages in negligence cases, several states have adopted comparative negligence statutes. For example, if the defendant's fault is found to be twice as great as that of the plaintiff, the latter will recover two-thirds of the damages and will be charged with the remainder of the loss (31, p. 436).

The following states have adopted comparative negligence statutes (quite frequently referred to as apportionment statutes): Mississippi, Georgia, Wisconsin, Nebraska, South Dakota, Arkansas, Maine, Hawaii, Massachusetts, Minnesota, New Hampshire, and Vermont (31, p. 437).

Actually, the apportionment statutes are not as clearly delineated as the example described previously (defendant two-thirds negligent, plaintiff one-third negligent) indicates. In Nebraska and South Dakota, the comparative negligence statute is limited to situations in which negligence of the plaintiff is slight, while that of the defendant is gross (31, p. 437). This type of application bars the doctrine of comparative negligence when the damages are anywhere near equal. Wisconsin, Georgia, Arkansas, Hawaii, Maine, Massachusetts, Minnesota, New Hampshire, and Vermont limit the doctrine to those cases where the plaintiff's negligence is not as great as that of the defendant (31, p. 437).

The apportionment of damages by comparing degrees of negligence has not had a widespread acceptance for several reasons. One reason is the lack of acceptance by members of the legal profession because comparative negligence can result in lower judgments for damages. Insurance companies have been known to oppose comparative negligence, because contributory negligence is no longer an absolute defense. Finally, the doctrine of comparative negligence is difficult to apply and becomes even more difficult when three or more parties are involved. Nevertheless, the doctrine does apply in a limited number of jurisdictions and, in those states, modifies the common law doctrine that contributory negligence is an absolute defense.

Statutes of Limitation

To limit the time in which a plaintiff can claim damages because of the breach of a legal duty by another, states have enacted statutes of limitation. These statutes fix the time in which an action may be brought. If the plaintiff fails to initiate a course of action within the time stipulated in the statute, the statute may be pleaded as an affirmative defense to the plaintiff's petition.

Normally, actions that are based on contractual agreements have a greater period of time in which they may be brought than do actions grounded in negligence and malpractice (16, Negligence, 1.18). Although the length of time varies from state to state, the usual limitations are two years for malpractice, three years for negligence, and four to five years for contractual agreements.

To compute the time limitation under a statute of limitation, the time at which the statute begins to run must be determined. Historically, the general rule has been that the statute begins to run from the date the breach of duty complained of occurred. In the case of malpractice, for example, the general rule has been that the statute commences to run from the time the wrongful act complained of occurred (16, Negligence 1.19). Several states, however, have adopted the discovery doctrine. In these jurisdictions, the statute does not begin to run until the wrongful act is discovered or, with reasonable diligence, should have been discovered (16, Negligence 1.20). This rule obviously is more liberal than the former rule and allows the complaining party more time in those cases in which the wrongful act could not have been discovered at the time it was committed. The discovery doctrine appears to be gaining favor. Fraudulent concealment of a wrongful act may also prevent the statute from running until such time as the fraud is discovered.

Contractual Relationships

Although this section is primarily devoted to the principles of liability normally associated with tort law (malpractice and negligence), several types of relationships which are essentially contractual are appropriately considered here. A contract is a promise or set of promises, the performance of which the law in some way recognizes as a duty and the breach of which the law provides a remedy for. Generally, the contractual agreement must be supported by consideration in order to be legally enforceable. Consideration is construed to be an act other than a promise, a forbearance, or a return promise which is bargained for (1, Section 1). Simply stated, consideration is something the parties to the contract bargain for, and the value is relatively unimportant. For example, it has been stated that a peppercorn will support consideration if it is the subject of bargaining.

Contractual relationships arise in a number of ways, many of which are quite routine. For example, a purchase of an article from a department store involves a contractual transaction known as a sale. The purchase of an airline ticket is contractual. Acceptance of employment is also a contractual relationship and may vary from a rather informal agreement to a very specific, well-defined set of duties and perogatives.

Contracts may be either oral or written, but certain types of contracts must be in writing to be enforceable. For example, a contract that is to be operative for a period longer than one year must be in writing to be enforceable; also, a written agreement involving the payment of money may, by statute, import a consideration merely because the agreement is in writing (23, Chapter 432.010, Section 7b).

As a very practical matter, most agreements that physical therapists and physical therapy schools enter into should be supported by a written contractual document that outlines in reasonable detail the rights, duties, and obligations of the parties involved. For example, a physical therapist providing consultative services to a health facility should, in the author's opinion, enter into a written agreement which would essentially contain provisions outlining the services to be performed, when the services are to be performed, the amount of services to be provided, the methods of payment for services rendered, a method of resolving any differences which might arise, and conditions for termination of the agreement.

Another type of contractual relationship is the agreement a physical therapy school enters into when it arranges with a clinical facility to provide clinical education for its students. Such an agreement should outline the school's responsibilities, the facility's responsibilities, and those areas which would normally be construed as joint responsibilities. The school's responsibilites might include but not necessarily be limited to the following items:

1. Provision of health and liability insurance for assigned students;
2. Designation and duties of the school's coordinator of clinical education;
3. Determination of student eligibility for assignment;
4. Types of information to be provided the clinical facility by the school;
5. Conditions for withdrawal of a student by the school;
6. Other areas which the school deems appropriate.

Examples of what might be included in the clinical facility's responsibilities are:

1. Designation and duties of the clinic's coordinator of clinical education;
2. Status of students (students or trainees-not employees);
3. Qualifications of clinical coordinator and instructors;
4. Appropriateness of facility (equipment, type of patient load, and so forth);
5. Emergency care of students (availability, cost, and so forth);
6. Conditions for withdrawal of a student at the request of the clinical facility;
7. Any other items which are deemed appropriate by the clinical facility.

Examples of areas which could be construed as joint responsibilities are:

1. Mutual determination of the objectives of clinical education;
2. Orientation of students to the policies, rules, and regulations of the clinical facility;
3. General conditions concerning the length of the contract, the method of termination, and any other conditions which the parties deem necessary.

A contractual relationship that has the potential of being a rather detailed instrument is one in which the physical therapist contracts to provide the entire physical therapy service for a health facility. The areas for consideration are many and varied. In this instance, the type of relationship desired by the parties will determine to a great extent many of the elements to be negotiated. Obviously the services to be provided will be enumerated along with methods of compensation, the purchase and maintenance of equipment, insurance, relationships to other departments, qualifications of personnel, methods of resolving differences which may arise and which are not specifically covered by the contract, and contract termination conditions. The foregoing are only a few examples of what such a contract would probably contain. Many other items would undoubtedly be considered.

Contractual relationships permeate all aspects of society. Contracts vary from simple oral and written agreements to highly complex instruments. When physical therapists enter into contractual relationships, they should use legal counsel familiar with the legal implications of contract law (particularly if the agreement is somewhat complex).

Malpractice Crisis

The application of the foregoing principles of liability to professional services and to health institutions created, beginning in the early 1970s, what has been commonly referred to as the *malpractice crisis*. The increasing number of negligence and malpractice claims filed, settled, and litigated; the rapidly rising cost of insurance protection; and the overall effect on the professions and the health institutions, in terms of risk and cost, created the crises.

Since the mid-1960s, the health care industry has been viewed as highly inflationary. The merits of this point of view have been subject to charge and countercharge and need not be debated in this chapter. It is sufficient to state that quality health care is expensive and that the malpractice crisis contributed significantly to the rapidly rising cost of insurance which became a cause of concern to many parties involved in the delivery of health services. Health professionals, hospitals, government (federal, state, local), and third party reimbursement agencies studied the problem, and various forms of action were undertaken in an effort to minimize the risk involved.

The Department of Health, Education, and Welfare between July 1 and October 31, 1976, analyzed about 4000 closed claims. These closed claims represented approximately 28 percent of the claims initiated in that year. The study revealed that 80 percent of the closed claims and 84 percent of the total dollars awarded were related to injuries that occurred in hospitals (46, p. 111-1). The most severe patient injuries were those caused by anesthesia and surgical error. Injuries caused by burns, falls, and so forth represented approximately 14 percent of the claims. Fortunately this latter category results in a relatively small number of serious injuries (46, p. 111-120.) Incident reports indicate that burns, falls, and equipment malfunctions are the most frequent causes of injuries that occur in physical therapy practice.

Legislative and Legal Responses

The several states responded to the malpractice crisis in various ways. During the period of 1975 and 1976, 43 states passed varying types of legislation designed to bring about some change in the tort system. For example, 36 states enacted legislation pertaining to the length of time stipulated in the statutes of limitation (46, p. V-1). The theory behind this type of legislation was based on a concept held by insurance companies that late discovered claims pose a particular problem for actuaries in trying to accurately determine malpractice insurance premiums (46, p. V-6). The effectiveness of this type of legislative change is not clear.

In addition to legislative changes that generally resulted in reducing the length of time in statutes of limitation, several states have experimented with other alternatives to the litigation process by implementing procedures for arbitration and for use of pretrial review or screening panels. State laws vary as to whether these measures are mandatory or voluntary.

Arbitration is used when the parties involved agree to arbitrate the claim and be bound by the results. This method has not been used extensively and its effectiveness is unclear. The evidence suggests that arbitrated cases reach conclusions more quickly, but it is not clear on whether arbitration reduces cost (46, p. V-2).

Pretrial screening or review panels (screening and review are used interchangeably) were initiated in an attempt to detect the bad, improper, and unjustified case from the case with merit and to allow only the latter to go to trial (25, p. 6). Although pretrial screening may be either voluntary or mandatory, most statutes allow the claimants to proceed to court if they so desire. Even with this provisio, several states have had their pretrial screening panels declared unconstitutional. Other states, however, have reached opposite conclusions and use these panels with varying results. The issues that involve constitutionality usually are concerned with "deprivation of the right to a jury" and denial of equal protection of the law. The later issue arises from the dispute over why there should be special legislation for providers of health care when similar protection is not given to the other professionals (25, p. 6). The effectiveness of pretrial screening is also open to question. Some of the evidence indicates that the awards are larger in those cases that have proceeded to trial following pretrial review. This may be caused by the fact that the less meritorious cases are either not pursued or are dropped because of pretrial requirements (46, p. V-3).

Modifications of Insurance Coverage

Prior to the escalation of medical malpractice and general liability insurance costs, providers generally purchased their coverage from commercial sources. The rapid increase in costs of insurance caused providers to explore alternative methods of protecting themselves and also at a reduced cost. The search for alternatives resulted in various approaches, from self-insurance and modification of deductibles to the development of limited-purpose insurance companies (often known as Captive Insurance Companies). The latter approach gained increasing acceptance by providers, particularly hospitals, as a mechanism to reduce the cost of malpractice and liability insurance.

The limited-purpose insurance companies were primarily sponsored by state and municipal hospital associations, investor owned hospital corporations, and, in some instances, groups of physicians. Growth of these companies has been quite rapid. As of October 1, 1979, there were 64 companies in operation—none of which existed prior to 1975 (21). The leading writers of medical malpractice insurance are still the well-established commercial companies, but the specialty companies have captured approximately 40 percent of the business (21).

In addition to the foregoing attempts to reduce the cost of insurance, providers, along with the expertise of the limited-purpose insurance companies, have been implementing *risk management programs*.

Risk Management

Health institutions for many years have to varying degrees operated safety programs. These programs, however, have generally confined their activities to employee and visitor safety. Very little was being accomplished in the area of malpractice. The malpractice crisis along with the efforts previously discussed gave rise to what is now commonly referred to as risk management. This term has generally been defined as "the identification, analysis and evaluation of risks and the selection of the most advantageous method for treating them" (36, p. 13). Unlike the traditional safety programs, risk management is a totally integrated program that combines all functions which may contribute to injury and subsequent monetary loss. To accomplish risk management, all personnel in health institutions must become more safety conscious. In other words, the implementation of a risk management program has to involve professionals and employees at all levels.

At the present time, hospitals are rapidly developing and implementing risk management programs and employing full time risk managers to direct and coordinate the various duties and aspects of the program. The key elements of a risk management program are:
1. Management involvement;
2. Risk management organization;
3. Incident reporting and investigation;
4. Inspections;
5. Communications (36, p. 14).

Without a doubt the area of risk management will continue to receive close attention in the future. Physical therapists practicing in hospitals will be involved in such programs. In addition, physical therapists will undoubtedly be involved in liability and malpractice studies because of the general belief that this area needs more data concerning what really constitutes a claim. Cost containment is an area of very high priority, and liability and malpractice losses are a contributing factor to increasing costs. Risk management may contribute to containing rapidly rising health care costs.

Summary and Recommendations

This section has discussed the laws pertaining to liability and malpractice along with a brief description of the legal elements involved in contractual relationships. Increasing litigation led to what has been generally referred to as the malpractice crisis. The efforts to alleviate the crisis have also been discussed, and practicing physical therapists undoubtedly will be involved in these efforts.

The following do's and don'ts are offered as practical and helpful recommendations to the reader:

Don'ts

1. Don't take on work for which you are not qualified.
2. Don't experiment.
3. Don't promise over optimistic results.
4. Don't delegate to unqualified people.
5. Don't criticize other physical therapists.
6. Don't panic if a complaint or accusation is made.
7. Don't admit fault.

The recommendation not to experiment deserves elaboration. The full statement should be: Don't experiment unless the protocol of what will be done has been well planned and properly approved and the informed consent of the patient(s) has been obtained.

Do's

1. Do make a thorough examination.
2. Do seek consultation when in doubt.
3. Do exercise tact.
4. Do watch your patient relationships.
5. Do check the condition of your equipment.
6. Do instruct patients carefully.
7. Do keep the referring physician informed.
8. Do make certain proper consent has been obtained.
9. Do select and supervise employees carefully.
10. Do keep good written records (24, pp. 114–119).

The maintenance of good written records is probably the most effective protection available to the physical therapist. Patients are inclined to remember every aspect of treatment but the professional who treats many patients is at a complete disadvantage when asked to recall specific details that occurred weeks, months, or even a year or two previously. Inadequate records can easily be construed to mean inadequate care. A good record not only indicates good care for the patient but in addition provides the best protection to the practicing physical therapist.

GOVERNMENTAL REQUIREMENTS

This section of the chapter discusses the legislation, most of which has been enacted within the last two decades, that imposes requirements on health care institutions and the professionals and employees who provide the health services. Legislation affecting reimbursement for services is beyond the scope of the section.

This section therefore is concerned with the requirements imposed by licensure and accreditation, workmen's compensation, and the National Labor Relations Act, Age Discrimination in Employment Act, and Rehabilitation Act. Although accreditation of health care institutions is essentially a voluntary system of evaluation and control, the requirements for accreditation have to a reasonable degree been recognized by legal authorities as having the force and effect of law. For this reason, accreditation has been included in this section on governmental requirements.

Licensure

The primary purpose of licensure (or registration in some states) is to protect the public from the unauthorized practice of the various professions. Licensure, therefore, when applied to physical therapy is designed to prevent unqualified individuals from holding themselves out to the public as being qualified to practice the profession. Not only does licensure protect the public and the profession from unauthorized practice, but it places requirements on individuals preparing to enter the profession. For example, certain educational requirements must be completed and in addition the candidate must successfully pass a licensure examination. Licensure also imposes, to a reasonable degree, minimum and maximum limitations on the right to practice.

Unlike the profession of medicine, which is considered to be a general profession and therefore has a wide range of authorized practice, physical therapy has been described as a limited profession; the limitation being that a physical therapist generally practices his or her profession under the referral from or orders of a licensed physician.

Scope of Activities

The scope of activities performed by limited professions has been gradually expanding. This expansion is probably the result of increasing reliance by physicians on the other health professionals, along with the increasing knowledge and skill of the latter. The scope of activities of physical therapists is experiencing the effect of this increase in reliance, knowledge, and skill. For example, the States of Maryland and California, and perhaps Nebraska, do not require physician referral in order for a physical therapist to undertake treatment. In addition, several states now allow the physical therapist to evaluate a patient without the requirement of referral from a physician. In fact, the official position of the American Physical Therapy Association (APTA) is that evaluation without physician referral should be generally recognized throughout the country (4). The author's opinion is that the profession of physical therapy, like other professions which have practiced under referral from the medical profession, will continue to gain a greater degree of independence. This gain, however, will place a greater legal responsibility on the profession, and the profession must meet this challenge. A primary method of meeting this challenge is for the profession to take steps to minimize the possibility that those individuals lacking the necessary knowledge and skill are allowed to practice. Establishing standards is one of these steps.

Standards

Evidence that the physical therapy profession has moved to establish standards of practice is found in an APTA publication that outlines and delineates "Standards of Physical Therapy Services" and "Standards for the Physical Therapy Practitioner." The two documents include not only the various standards but interpretations of those standards. The former is accompanied by an evaluation form that can be used to evaluate the physical therapy service, and the latter includes standards on a wide range of individual practitioner obligations, from personal qualities and ethical conduct to consultation and community responsibility. The frequent updating and revision of these standards, since their original adoption in 1971 and 1972, reflects the expanding scope of activities of the physical therapist (2).

These standards provide a method by which the profession can measure optimal performance, and they represent the heart of a profession—service to society. Further, standards such as these can be expected to affect licensure requirements and preparation for entry into the profession.

Accreditation

Organizations that accredit various components of health care are many and varied. Most pertinent, however, is the Joint Commission on Accreditation of Hospitals (JCAH). The JCAH is a voluntary organization which historically has made its services available to mental health and extended care facilities. Although the JCAH as previously indicated is a voluntary agency, approval by the JCAH has been accepted by federal authorities as meeting the criteria for hospital participation in the Medicare-Medicaid Program, and to that extent its activities have the force and effect of law.

The JCAH under the title of Rehabilitation Program Services devotes one standard to physical therapy. Essentially this standard states that the program shall be under the direction of a qualified physical therapist who is a graduate of an accredited school, who has demonstrated competence, and who has met the legal requirements of licensure. Staff physical therapists shall have met the required educational requirements and also shall be legally licensed. In addition, sufficient supervision must be provided to individual personnel (20, pp. 165–166). The standards adopted by the APTA not only meet but in all probability exceed the standards of the JCAH.

Workmen's Compensation

The first section of this chapter concentrated on the legal implications that arise as the result of negligence and malpractice. These are conditions wherein a patient or a visitor is the individual who has claimed harm. Thus far this chapter has not mentioned injuries to employees. Physical therapists, and particularly those that practice as independent contractors, do, however, employ individuals to assist them in their practice. It is not unusual for employees to incur injuries arising out of and in the course of employment.

Prior to the passage of the Workmen's Compensation Act, certain common law defenses were open to the employer when an employee suffered an injury while acting within the scope of his or her employment. The primary defenses were:

1. The employee was injured as the result of the negligence of a fellow servant or employee.
2. The employee assumed the risk of the position.
3. The employee was injured as a result of his own negligence.

Understandably, with these defenses available to an employer, many of the injuries sustained by employees resulted in no liability on the part of the employers and no duty to compensate the employees for their injuries.

Statutes

With the passage of the Workmen's Compensation statutes, the common law defenses were abolished. The major test of an employer's liability for an injury sustained by an employee is determined primarily by the answer to the following question: "Did the injury complained of arise out of and in the course of the employment'" If the answer to the foregoing question is yes, the employee's injury is generally considered to compensable.

Workmen's Compensation statutes vary from state to state, although the legal principles are quite similar. Missouri, for example, differentiates between a major and minor employer, a major employer being defined as an employer who regularly has more than 10 employees. A minor employer is defined as an employer who regularly employs 10 or less employees (23, Section 287.050).

Minor employers generally have the right to reject the Workmen's Compensation Act unless the employment is construed to be hazardous. If an employer rejects the Act, he or she may not then assert the common law defenses previously enumerated if an injured employee initiates claim (40). The common law defenses are available to the employer, however, if the employee elects to reject the Act (41, Section 187.080).

As a general rule, however, liability for an injury to an employee, as previously indicated, revolves primarily around the issue: "Did the injury complained of arise out of and in the course of employment?" Brief examples are cited to illustrate the legal interpretation of this question.

1. A female employee who had just returned to work after lunch started to sit down in the lounge to apply cosmetics and, because the chair had been moved by another employee, sat on the floor, injuring herself; it was determined that her injury arose out of and in the course of her employment (6).
2. A "utility butcher," arriving at work at least one hour before he was due to start work, began sharpening knives, an operation which could have been done during regular hours, and sustained an injury while so

engaged; the accident was construed to have arisen out of and in the course of his employment (17).

3. A filling station manager, returning to work from his house 15 miles away, where he had delivered kerosene during his lunch hours was injured in a collision with a train while driving his own truck; it was held in this case that he was not injured during and in the course of his employment (17).

Although the employer is liable irrespective of negligence, willful failure of an employee to use safety devices provided by the employer—provided the employer has made a diligent effort to cause the employee to use the safety device—can relieve the employer of liability. Also, compensation will be denied for self-inflicted injury, but the burden of proof of intentional self-inflicted injury is placed on the employer.

National Labor Relations Act

The National Labor Relationships Act (NLRA) was originally enacted in 1935, It was subsequently amended in 1947 (Taft-Hartley) and by the Labor Management and Disclosure Act of 1959. Until 1974 the act excluded not-for-profit hospitals. The law specifically excluded "Corporations or Associations operating a hospital if no part of the net earnings inure to the benefit of any private shareholder or individual" (26, Section 2(2)).

In August 1974, Congress enacted Public Law 93-360, which removed the exclusion of not-for-profit hospitals from the NLRA. Congress also defined what shall constitute a health care institution. The 1974 amendment states that a "health care institution" shall include "any hospital, health maintenance organization, health clinic, nursing home, extended care facility, or other institution devoted to the care of the sick, infirm, or aged person" (26, Section 2 (14)).

The NLRA applies to organizaions that are construed to be engaged in interstate commerce. From a very practical point of view, most health organizations under standards established by the National Labor Relations Board (the administering agency) will be construed to be engaged in interstate commerce and subject to the Act's provisions.

State and federal employees are excluded from the provision of the NLRA; however, federal employees may organize and bargain collectively under Executive Order 11491 as amended. The right of state, county, and municipal employees to organize is governed by state and local laws, and the laws pertaining thereto vary rather widely.

The NLRA assures employees of the right to self-organization, to form, join, or assist labor organizations to bargain collectively through representatives of their own choosing and to engage in other concerted activities for the purpose of collective bargaining or other mutual aid or protection, as well as the right to refrain from the above (26, Section 7).

Unfair Practices

The act provides that certain practices by employers and employees constitute unfair labor practices and are therefore unlawful. Briefly, unfair labor practices on the part of an employer are as follows:

1. Illegal interference, restraint, and coercion (26, Section 8(a)(1));
2. Illegal assistance or domination (26, Section 8(a)(2));
3. Discrimination to encourage or discourage union activity (26, Section 8(a)(3));
4. Discrimination for filing charges or giving testimony (26, Section 8 (a)(4));
5. Refusal to bargain collectively (26, Section 8(a)(5)).

Union unfair labor practices are briefly enumerated below:

1. Union restraint and coercion (26, Section 8(a)(1)(A)(B));
2. Union discrimination (26, Section 8(b)(3));
3. Union refusal to bargain (26, Section 8(b)(3));
4. Secondary boycotts (26, Section 8(b)(4));
5. Excessive initiation fees (26, Section 8(b)(5));
6. Featherbedding (26, Section 8(b)(6));
7. Certain types of organizational and recognitional picketing (26, Section 9(b)(7));
8. Hot cargo agreements (26, Section 8(b)(e)).

Bargaining

The heart of labor management relations is collective bargaining, and the failure to bargain in good faith is an unfair practice for both labor and managment. The subjects of collective bargaining are *wages, hours, and conditions of employment* (26, Section 8(b)(7)(d)). This has been construed to include a vast array of activities such as insurance, pensions, overtime, layoff, and recall and many other areas which are related to wages, hours and conditions of employment.

When Congress was considering the 1974 amendments to the NLRA, concern was expressed that work interruptions could jeopardize the health and well-being of patients. In an effort to at least minimize this potential, Congress provided that a labor organization must give 90 days notice of its intent to renegotiate an existing contract instead of the 60 days required of other organizations (26, Section 8 (b)(d)(A)). Where the bargaining is for an initial contract, 30 days notice of the existence of a dispute must be given to the Federal Mediation and Conciliation Service (26, Section 8(b)(d)(B)). Both labor and management are required to participate fully with the Concilliation Service (26, Section 8(b)(d)(C)). In addition, the amendment requires a labor organization to give 10 days notice of its intent to engage in a strike, picketing, or other concerted refusal to work (26, Section (8)(B)(g)). Whether these efforts by Congress to minimize work stoppages have been effective is open to question. Work stoppages appear to be less in health institutions (5 percent) than in other institutions (13 percent), but these figures are deceptive and merit additional study (47, p. 321).

In addition to the foregoing amendments pertaining to health care institutions, one other amendment refers to members of religious groups whose tenets or teachings contain objections to joining and/or supporting union organizations. This provision allows such an individual, in lieu of paying periodic dues, to make a like contribution to an organization exempt from taxation under the Internal Revenue Code (26, Section 19).

Bargaining Units

Prior to the 1974 amendments, legislation pertaining to labor relations that applied to not-for-profit hospitals was limited to action by the various states. Fourteen states had varying types of labor relations legislation which to some extent followed the provisions of the NLRA. The federal law provides that, for the purposes of collective bargaining, employees shall be assigned to appropriate bargaining units (26, Section 9(a)). The state agencies responsible for the administration of the state labor laws were most liberal in interpreting what constituted appropriate units, and this resulted in a proliferation of bargaining units. Management, in turn, was required to bargain with a multiplicity of units which had the tendency to increase instability in labor management relations.

The criteria generally applied to determine the appropriateness of a unit were (and are) to be:

1. Similarity of skills;
2. History of collective bargaining;
3. Desires of employees.

In considering the 1974 NLRA amendments to minimize instability, Congress indicated that their intent was to avoid the proliferation of bargaining units and cautioned the National Labor Relations Board (NLRB) concerning this issue. As might be expected, the initial questions that required determination concerned the appropriateness of bargaining units in not-for-profit hospitals.

The question reached the NLRB in 1975. The NLRB, noting the reports of the Senate and House Committees on preventing proliferation of bargaining units, determined the following five units to be appropriate:

1. Registered nurses;
2. All other professionals;
3. Technical employees;
4. Clerical employees in business offices;
5. Service and maintenance employees.

In 1977, the NLRB added a sixth unit: Employee physicians. This unit excluded House Staff (47, p. 395-6).

On examination of the above named units, it appears that physical therapists would be included in "All other professionals." In a health care institution, this unit would probably include dietitians, pharmacists, medical record librarians, occupational therapists, and other individuals who meet the definition of a professional.

Solicitation

Another area that has generated a considerable amount of legal interpretation concerns union solicitation by employees. Health care institutions generally promulgate rules and regulations concerning solicitation and distribution of literature by employees. The NLRB took the position that employee solicitation must be allowed during nonwork time and in areas which would not effect patient care. Two cases involving this issue have resulted in U.S. Supreme Court decisions.

The first case (the Beth Israel case) involved solicitation in the hospital cafeteria. The Court held that solicitation in the cafeteria could not be banned when less than 20 percent of the patrons were patients (5).

While the Beth Israel case involved only the cafeteria, the second case to reach the Supreme Court involved other areas of the hospital. The Court concluded that solicitation could be banned in patient corridors, patient floors, sitting rooms, and immediate patient care areas. The Court let stand the NLRB's ruling that the hospital could not ban solicitation in such areas as the gift shop, cafeteria, and first floor corridors (28). As a result of these decisions, the NLRB General Counsel has issued guidelines that essentially conform to the foregoing decisions (29).

Results and Implications

The intent of Congress in adopting the 1974 NLRA amendments was to provide for collective bargaining in the health care field and to provide procedures to promote the peaceful resolution of disputes. Attempts to organize the unorganized in health care institutions have increased. The "win rate" for unions has been approximately 60 percent, but this is expected to decrease to approximately the national average of about 50 percent (47). Work interruptions have probably increased to some extent, but not to the degree predicted by opponents of the amendments.

Physical therapists employed by health care institutions are now within the purview of the National Labor Relations Act. Whether they are employees under the Act or representatives of management, physical therapists must conform to the laws, rules, and regulations pertaining to labor management relations if organization is to occur in their work settings.

Fair Labor Standards Act

In 1938 Congress enacted the Fair Labor Standards Act (FLSA) (45, S. 21). In 1963, the "Equal Pay" amendment was added to the Act, and in 1967 the Act was again amended to bring most hospitals under its purview. The legislation is administered by the Department of Labor, with the exception of the equal pay provisions, which were transferred to the Equal Employment Opportunity Commission. The FLSA has many and varied ramifications but its main features consist of the following:

1. Establishes a minimum wage;
2. Established the maximum hours that can be worked without payment of overtime;
3. Prohibits wage discrimination based on sex; and
4. Prohibits child labor.

The 1967 amendment to the FLSA extended coverage, with certain exemptions, to all nongovernmental hospital employees; in 1974 this coverage was extended to employees of state and local governments. The U.S. Supreme Court in 1976 ruled, however, that such coverage was in violation of the Tenth Amendment, and this decision removed state and local government employees from the Act's provisions (27).

Exemptions

The FLSA does not cover all employees in a health care institution. Volunteers, for example, are not covered because no employment relationship exists. In addition, students and independent contractors are exempt. Trainees in health care organizations are generally exempt if: 1) the training is similar to that given in a vocational school; 2) the training is for the benefit of the trainee or student; 3) the trainee or student does not displace a regular employee; 4) the employer who provides the training derives no immediate advantage; 5) the trainees or students are not necessarily entitled to positions at the completion of the training period; and 6) employers and the trainees or students are not entitled to wages for the time spent in training (39, p. 8:2). Physical therapy students in clinical education would seem to be within this exemption, as would medical students pursuing clinical training in a hospital. In addition to the foregoing, the FLSA exempts those who are employed in an executive, administrative, or professional capacity.

Executive and Administrative Employees

An executive is defined as any employee:
1. Whose primary duty consists of the management of the enterprise;
2. Who customarily and regularly directs the work of two or more persons;
3. Who has the right to hire and fire or to recommend such action;
4. Who customarily and regularly exercises discretion;
5. Who, in the case of a hospital, does not devote as much as 40 percent of his or her hours of work time per week to activities which are not directly related to the activities enumerated in items 1 through 4; and,
6. Who is paid at a rate of not less than $155 per week.
   If an employee is compensated at a rate of not less than $250 per week and performs management functions, the so-called simplified test applies

and he shall be deemed to meet the requirements of an executive (44, S. 541.1).

The performance of management functions includes interviewing, selecting and training, setting hours and rates of pay, directing the work of others, maintaining supervisory records, approving performance, adjusting grievances, disciplining, and apportioning work (44, S. 541.102(b)). An administrative employee may be exempt from the FLSA if the primary duty consists of nonmanual work that is directly related to management or general business policies of the employer or the employer's customers. This exemption also includes an administrative employee who regularly exercises discretion and independent judgment and in addition regularly assists an executive or administrator, handles special assignments, and performs technical or specialized work under general supervision (44, S. 541.2). Administrative employees must also be paid not less than $155 per week. If remunerated at not less than $250 per week, the simplified test applicable to executives will also apply to administrative employees (44, S. 541.2).

The FLSA regulations also exempt employees who qualify as professionals. A professional is an individual whose primary duty meets one or more of the following criteria:

1. Work that requires knowledge of an advanced type in a field of science or learning;
2. Work that is original or creative in character in a recognized field of artistic endeavor;
3. Teaching, training, or tutoring. In addition, a professional employee must exercise discretion and judgment and must perform work that is predominantly intellectual and varied in character. A professional employee must not devote more than 20 percent of his time to work not essentially professional in character and must be remunerated at not less than $170 per week (44, S. 541.3).

Employees who meet the foregoing definitions and criteria are exempt from the provisions of the FLSA and from the following requirements pertaining to work week, working time, and minimum wage.

Work Week

The FLSA provides that an employer shall not require an employee to work more than 40 hours per week without the payment of overtime for hours worked in excess of 40. Overtime is to be computed at one and one-half times the regular rate (10, S. 760-(1)). Where the 40-hour week is used, overtime need not be paid for hours in excess of eight per day. Hospitals, however, have been granted an exception that allows them to compute overtime based on 80 hours incurred during a 14-day period. The provision requires that the employer and employee must mutually agree to this exception prior to the performance of any work. When this exception is used, the hospital must pay overtime for any hours in excess of 80 during the 14-day period. The hospital is under no obligation to offer this exception and need not offer it to all employees. If an employee rejects this exception, the 40-hour work week applies (45, S. 207 (J) as amended).

Working Time

Questions concerning what constitutes working hours will naturally continue to arise from time to time, but the following categories have generally been construed to constitute (with certain noted exceptions) hours worked.

Rest and Meal Time. Coffee breaks and short rest periods are considered to be working time. Meal periods generally are not hours worked if the time allowed is at least 30 minutes and the employee is completely relieved from duty (39, 8:6).

Sleeping Time. "Employees who are required to be on duty for less than 24 hours are considered to be on working time even if they are permitted to sleep or perform personal activities when not busy. For example, telephone operators who nap between calls are still on 'working time' if such naps are permitted. If the period is greater than 24 hours, the employer and employee may agree to exclude from working time bonafide meal periods and a scheduled sleeping period not to exceed eight hours, provided adequate sleeping conditions are furnished by the employer and the employee can usually enjoy an uninterrupted nights sleep" (39, 8:7).

Lectures, Meetings, and Training Programs. Attendance at activities of this type is considered to be working time unless the following criteria are all complied with:

1. Attendance is outside regular working hours;
2. Attendance is voluntary;
3. The activity is not directly related to the employee's job; and
4. No productive work is performed (39, 8:7).

Travel Time. Normally, travel time to and from work is not considered to be working time. Travel during the workday constitutes hours worked. Travel to another location to perform emergency work after completing a normal day's work is compensable. There are, however, various exceptions to this category (39, 8:8).

Waiting Time. Idle time which occurs during the normal duty time is generally construed to be time worked (39, 8:6). The general rule is that any work which the employer has permitted is working time. The burden is placed on the employer to make certain that work is not performed unless the employer wants it to be.

Overtime. Overtime is defined as hours worked in excess of 40 when a 40-hour work week is being observed. A health care institution, as previously indicated, may elect with the employee's acceptance to use the exception of an 80-hour work period. This exception requires overtime pay for hours worked in excess of eight per day and in excess of 80 in 14-day period.

Overtime pay for hours worked in excess of eight hours per day may be credited to overtime for hours worked in excess of 80 per 14-day period (39, 8:10). The overtime rate is computed at one and one-half times the regular hourly rate of pay. This overtime computation applies even though the employee is salaried but is not exempt from the FLSA. The regular rate includes such things as shift differentials but does not include gifts, vacations, pensions, and benefits such as profit sharing. Compensatory time may be granted in lieu of monetary payment for overtime but it must be granted during the same pay period in which it was earned and at the rate of one and one-half times the number of overtime hours worked (39, 8:10-11-13).

Minimum Wage

Effective January 1, 1980, the minimum hourly wage rate for employees subject to the FLSA was increased from $2.90 per hour to $3.10 per hour. On January 1, 1981, this rate will be increased to $3.35 per hour. Certain categories of employees may be employed at subminimum rates by special certification. These categories include student learners who are employed on a part-time basis pursuant to a training program at an accredited school, as well as full-time students, handicapped workers, and apprentices (39, 8:16–17).

A patient worker is an aged, sick, or mentally ill individual who receives treatment or care by a hospital whether he or she is resident or not and who has an employment relationship with the institution (39, 8:18). The test of whether an employment relationship exists will be determined largely on whether the work is of any economic benefit. Its therapeutic value does not enter into the determination (39, 8:18).

Required Records

Enforcement of the FLSA requires that the employer keep and maintain certain records in order for representatives of the federal government to determine if a violation has or has not been committed (45, S. 211 (c)). Records which must be kept on each employee include the following: 1) name and employee number; 2) home address; 3) date of birth if under 19; 4) sex and occupation; 5) time of day and day of week that the employee's work week begins; 6) regular hourly rate of pay for any week in which overtime is worked, overtime compensation due, basis on which wages are paid, and the amount and kind of payment which is excluded; 7) hours worked each work day, and the total each work week; 8) total daily or straight time earnings; 9) total overtime compensation; 10) additions or deductions from wages for each pay period; 11) total compensation each pay day; and 12) payment date and pay period covered (44, S. 516.2). The above records must be available for inspection.

Collective bargaining agreements, special exceptions to overtime standards, and payroll records along with the usual business records showing dollar volume must be kept for three years (44, S. 516.5).

Basic time and earning sheets, wage rate tables, work schedules, usual record of invoices, billings to patients, and additions to and deductions from wages paid along with records which explain the basis for any wage differential between the sexes must be maintained for a period of two years (44, S. 516.6). Where a health institution has elected to use the 14-day work period, records supporting this election must also be maintained (44, S. 516.23).

Child Labor

The provision in the FLSA pertaining to child labor was directed toward oppressive child labor practices. In general, this provision prohibits hiring individuals under the age of 16 years unless the employer is the parent or guardian of the child, and only if the employment is construed not to be a hazardous occupation as determined by the Secretary of Labor. Employers who provide employment in hazardous occupations may employ workers between the ages of 16 and 18 years. Children between the ages of 14 and 16 years may be employed in nonhazardous activity if the hours do not interfere with schooling, health, and well-being. As a general rule, it is a good practice to obtain proof of age in questionable cases (39, 8:19).

Equal Pay Act

The Equal Pay Act (EPA) of 1963 has had a significant effect on health care institutions because of the large number of female employees. Passed as an amendment to the Fair Labor Standards Act (FLSA), the EPA was enacted to correct differing rates of pay for male and female employees when the work demands of the position are equal. In short, equal work requires equal pay. "Equal work" is generally defined as work that requires "equal skill, effort and responsibility and which is performed under similar working conditions" (39, 9:31).

The EPA applies to all employees covered by the minimum wage law. Although the U.S. Supreme Court has held (as indicated earlier) that the minimum wage and overtime provisions of the FLSA do not apply to state and local government employees, the federal courts have held that the equal pay provisions of the EPA do apply to these employees and are not unconstitutional (39, 9:31). In addition, by virtue of a 1972 amendment, equal pay coverage was extended to include executive, administrative, and professional personnel (39, 9:36). This, of course, has the effect of extending equal pay coverage to the employees who generally occupy higher paid positions. As an amendment to the FLSA, the EPA is enforced by the Wage and Hour Division of the Department of Labor.

Equal Work

Although the purpose of the Act (as previously noted) is to eliminate pay differences based on sex when the work is equal, courts have struggled with the question of "What constitutes equal work?" As a result "equal work" has been construed as identical at one extreme and comparable or similar at the other extreme (39, 9:32).

Equal skill takes into consideration such factors as experience, training, and ability. Equal effort is concerned with the degree of physical or mental exertion needed for the job. Equal responsibility is directed toward the degree of accountability that performance in the position requires. Similar working conditions, as the term is used, implies a flexible standard, so jobs in different departments could be construed as having similar working conditions (39, 9:32-33).

Implications

In the health care industry, most of the questions about equal pay have been concerned with aides, orderlies, and maids and porters. Generally higher pay for male orderlies has been asserted by health care employers on the basis of duties that require strength, as in lifting and transporting patients. The strength required has also been claimed to justify higher pay for porters (males) than for maids (females). In the final analysis, however, each situation is decided on its own merits. Differentials in pay that are based on physical effort are allowable, but the employer must be able to demonstrate that this physical effort is primary to the position and not merely incidental. Equally vital is the need to make certain that these more difficult tasks are not performed by employees who are not compensated to perform them (39, 9:34).

The employer has the burden of proving that wage differentials are not based on sex. The employer may also show that wage differentials are based on seniority, merit, or quantity or quality of work. A wage differential paid to an employee who is the head of a household is invalid (39, 9:35).

An employer found to be in violation of the EPA may be liable for such things as back pay based on the unjustified differential and damages in an amount equal to the back pay plus attorneys' fees and interest (39, 9:36).

The Equal Pay Act makes it most important that individuals who participate in the preparation of job descriptions exercise great care in describing positions in which the skills, efforts, and responsibilities are similar and for which both males and females are or can be employed.

Civil Rights Act

Some form of civil rights legislation has been in effect since 1866 but it was not until 1964 that major legislation was enacted with the primary purpose of eliminating discrimination in employment and other conditions. Title VII of the Civil Rights Act of 1964 prohibits an employer who employs 15 or more persons in an industry affecting commerce from discriminating against job applicants and employees because of race, color, sex, religion or national origin (11, S. 2000e). The act is enforced by the Equal Employment Opportunity Commission.

Unlawful Practices

The most pertinent sections of Title VII pertaining to employers and employees are sections 703(a) and 703(d), which make it an unlawful employment practice for an employer to:

1. Fail or refuse to hire or to discharge any individual or otherwise to discriminate against any individual with respect to his compensation, terms, conditions, or privileges of employment because of such individual's race, color, sex, religion, or national origin; or
2. Limit, segregate, or classify employees or applicants for employment in any way that would deprive or tend to deprive any individual of employment opportunities or otherwise adversely affect his status as an employee, because of such individual's race, color, sex, religion, or national origin.

Section 703 (d) also makes it unlawful for any employer, labor organization, or joint labor management committee controlling apprenticeship, or other type of training, to discriminate in regard to admission to such programs.

Other practices that have been made unlawful are:

1. Discriminating against an employee who has filed charges;
2. Advertising in a manner that tends to discriminate because of race, color, sex, religion, or national origin; and
3. Discriminating in hiring, dismissal, promotion, or tenure because of pregnancy.

The primary purpose of the Civil Rights Act was to eliminate discrimination in employment based on race or color. Initially, this area received the most attention but in recent years discrimination based on sex has been receiving increasing attention along with religion, the latter, however, to a lesser degree than sex.

Race or Color

Title VII of the Civil Rights Act prohibits discriminatory practices in recruiting, hiring, promotion, discharge, and other benefits where such practices can be construed as based on race or color. Refusing to hire a black employee who answered in the affirmative on an application form as to whether he had ever been arrested has been held to be a violation. The court has also held, however, that no discrimination occurred when a black employee was discharged after the employer discovered the extent of the employee's prior criminal record for theft and receiving stolen goods. Other employment practices that have been held to be discriminatory more against black than white include:

1. Consideration of an individual's poor credit rating;
2. Discharge because the employee's wages were garnished;
3. Consideration of the fact that a woman is an unwed mother;
4. Requirement of a high school diploma;
5. Prohibition of Afro hair style (39, (39, 9:5).

Sex

As indicated previously, discrimination based on sex has been receiving considerable attention in recent years. Title VII of the Civil Rights Act does not limit discrimination based on sex to women. The Act also applies to men who have been denied employment to positions essentially construed to be "women's jobs." One exception exists to the general prohibition of discrimination on grounds of sex, religion, or national origin, and that exception pertains to those instances where the foregoing characteristics constitute a bonafide occupational qualification (BFOQ) reasonably necessary to the normal operation of the particular business or enterprise (11, S. 2000 (c), Title VII, Section 703 (e)(1)). However, the Equal Employment Opportunity Commission has indicated that the BFOQ exception will be narrowly construed (11, S. 1604 (2)(a)). Thus, it has been held a violation to refuse an application of a male licensed vocational nurse in a nursing home where 75 percent of its patients were female. A policy not to hire a female who has preschool age children while hiring men who have preschoolers is a violation. Fringe benefits such as medical, hospital, accident, and life insurance must be granted equally to men and women.

Pregnancy and Maternity

Policies relating to pregnancy have also received attention. For example, loss of seniority because of pregnancy has been held to be violative (39, 9:12-13). In 1978, Congress, in an effort to prevent discrimination in employment because of pregnancy, amended Title VII (33). As a result, an employer who fails to hire and promote or who discharges a woman solely because of pregnancy is in violation of the act. Employers are not required to provide special conditions for pregnant employees but must treat pregnant workers the same as any other employee.

Maternity benefits have also received attention. Legislation was enacted in 1978 to prohibit discrimination based on pregnancy and to provide that pregnancy be treated as any other temporary disability (32).

Religion

Discrimination based on religion has raised very few issues when compared with discrimination based on race and sex. Title VII of the Civil Rights Act states that the term "religion" includes all aspects of religious observance and practice as well as belief. Discrimination based on religion is a violation unless an employer demonstrates that he is unable to reasonably accommodate to an employee's or prospective employee's religious observance or practice without undue hardship on the conduct of the employer's business (42, Section 701 (J)). An exception may also be made for a bonafide occupational qualification.

Title VII does not clearly define religion but court cases have generally agreed that it is a "sincere and meaningful belief which occupies in the life of its possessor a place parallel to that filled by the God" of traditional religions. Atheism, if it is an employee's sincerely held belief, may be included under the term religion (39, 9:17). A case recently decided by the U.S. Supreme Court involved the requirement that an employee work on Saturday, the day on which the employee's religion observed religious services. The Court held that an accommodation was not absolutely required because this would deprive other employees of their rights under the act (43).

National Origin

Discrimination based on national origin, like that based on religion, has received little attention. Discrimination on this basis is obviously unlawful unless an employer can demonstrate a bonafide occupational qualification. Discharge of an employee because of heavily accented English has been held to be discriminatory. Refusing to allow Spanish speaking people to speak Spanish on the job has also been held to be discriminatory (39, 9:19).

Seniority, Merit, and Selection

An employer is permitted to maintain and apply different standards of compensation, or different terms, conditions, or privileges of employment pursuant to a bonafide seniority or merit system, provided that such differences are not the result of an intention to discriminate because of race, color, sex, religion, or national origin (42, Section 703 (n)).

Section 703(h) of Title VII also provides that it shall not be an unlawful employment practice for an employer to give and to act upon the results of any professionally developed ability test provided that such test is not designed to discriminate because of race, color, sex, religion, or national origin. The Supreme Court has held that if a test has a discriminatory effect, the employer must demonstrate that the use of the test is required by business necessity and that the test is related to job performance. Even though the employer has no intent to discriminate, that alone is not sufficient to validate the use of tests which have the effect of excluding racial or other minorities protected by Title VII (15).

Over the years, as expected, a great amount of conflict has occurred over the interpretation of lawful and unlawful employee selection procedures. The four federal equal employment opportunity agencies, the Departments of Labor and Justice, the Equal Employment Opportunity Commission, and the U.S. Civil Service Commission in 1978 published the *Uniform Guidelines on Employee Selection Procedures*. These guidelines are intended to establish a uniform position for determining whether employment practices discriminate on grounds of race, color, sex, religion, or national origin. The guidelines became effective September 25, 1978.

Enforcement and Remedy

As previously indicated, the Equal Employment Opportunity Commission (EEOC) is the enforcement agency. This agency will, however, defer to state agencies in many instances if state law is similar to federal law. Where a violation is alleged, the EEOC may bring an action against an employer, or if the EEOC chooses not to act, the employee is not precluded from maintaining a separate legal action on his or her own behalf. Remedies that are available to correct discriminatory practice include reinstatement, back pay, injunctive relief, affirmative action, payment of attorneys' fees, and, in aggravated cases, compensatory and punitive damage (39, 9:26-27-28-29).

Age Discrimination in Employment Act

The Age Discrimination in Employment Act (ADEA), enacted by Congress in 1967, prohibits age discrimination by an employer who employs 20 or more persons in an industry affecting commerce. The Act's purpose is to promote the employment of older persons based on their ability rather than age (39, 9:31). In 1974, the ADEA was amended in order to place federal, state, and local governments and their agencies on the list of employers subject to the Act (39, 9:39).

Originally the ADEA applied to individuals who were at 40 and less than 65 years of age. In 1978 Congress again amended the act, the primary purpose being to raise the upper age limit to 70 years of age. The 1978 amendments became effective January 1, 1979 (39, 9:39). The essential features of the 1978 amendments are as follows:

1. Mandatory retirement based on age is prohibited prior to age 70.
2. Employees covered by a collective bargaining agreement which was in effect on September 1, 1977 were not affected by the act until termination of the contract or on January 1, 1980, whichever was first.
3. The amendments were not applicable to employees in the 65–70 age category who had been terminated or forced to retire prior to the effective date of the amendments (39, 9:29).

The ADEA continues to make it unlawful for an employer:

1. "To fail or refuse to hire or to discharge any individual or otherwise discriminate against any individual with respect to his compensation, terms, conditions, or privileges of employment, because of such individual's age;
2. "To limit, segregate, or classify employees in any way which would deprive or tend to deprive any individual of employment opportunities or otherwise adversely affect his status as an employee because of such individual's age;
3. "To reduce the wage rate of any employee in order to comply with this act" (45, S. 623 (a)).

A health institution may, however, take any action otherwise prohibited by the Act when,

1. Age is a bonafide occupational qualification and is reasonably necessary for normal operations of the business;
2. Differentiations are made on reasonable factors other than age;

3. Differentiation is based on a bonafide seniority system or employee benefit plan;
4. An individual is disciplined or discharged for cause (16, Vol. II-5-2).

It has also been held that The Age Discrimination Act is applicable to advertising that indicates age preference. For example, notices that contain phrases such as "young" "age 25 to 35," "recent college graduate," "supplement your pension," and so forth, have been construed as discriminatory (39, 9:39).

The Act does, however, allow for certain exceptions, which are enumerated above. For example, when age limitation are imposed by law or regulation, this is a bonafide occupational qualification (39, 9:38). An employer may also use the results of validated employee tests to make employment decisions but the tests must be specifically related to the requirements of the position (39, 9:40).

As indicated previously, employers who have more than 20 employees are subject to the ADEA. Physical therapists operating their own organizations could be affected by the law. Physical therapists employed by health organizations should be aware of the Act and its implications. The remedies that are available to an individual who claims discrimination based on age include the right to sue for the amount alleged to have been lost as the result of the discrimination. Reinstatement, if an employee's job has been lost, is another remedy that is available.

Rehabilitation Act

In 1973 Congress, in an effort to eliminate discriminatory practices involving the handicapped, enacted the Rehabilitation Act of 1973 (45, Section 794). The two pertinent sections of this Act are Sections 503 and 504.

Section 503 of the Rehabilitation Act applies to government contractors whose contracts are in excess of $2,500 and requires that such contractors must prepare an affirmative action plan which is applicable to handicapped employees. Contractors who hold contracts in excess of $50,000 must put such a plan in writing (39, 9:55). Section 503 is administered and enforced by the Department of Labor. This section could have applicability to physical therapists who contract to provice services for government agencies.

Section 504 provides that no otherwise qualified handicapped individual in the United States shall, solely by reasons of his or her handicap, be excluded from participation in, or be denied benefit of, or be subjected to discrimination under any program or activity receiving federal financial assistance (35, Section 504). Administration of Section 504 has been delegated to the U.S. Department of Health, Education and Welfare, now the U.S. Department of Health and Human Services.

There has been some confusion as to whom Section 504 applies. The administering agency, however, has by regulation taken the position that the law applies to institutions which receive Medicare, Medicaid, Hill-Burton or other federal support. For purposes of this section, the regulations—although questioned by some legal authorities—will be presumed to be applicable to all health care institutions.

Handicapped Person

The regulations define a "handicapped person" as an individual who has a physical or mental impairment that substantially limits one or more major life activities, who has a record of such impairment, or who is regarded as having such an impairment. The foregoing regulation has been interpreted to include alcoholics and drug addicts. The regulations provide, however, that only qualified handicapped persons are protected by the law and thus alcoholics and addicts whose handicaps might impede their job performance may be treated as unqualified (39, 9:56). A qualified handicapped person is defined as one who, with reasonable accommodations, can perform the essential functions of the job in question. Thus, an employer may not insist that a handicapped perform all aspects of the job—only those that are essential (39, 9:57).

Employer Obligations

The purpose of the Rehabilitation Act is to prevent employment practices that could be construed as discriminatory against a qualified handicapped person solely because of the handicap. In addition, the law imposes on employers an obligation to take positive steps to hire and promote qualified handicapped individuals (39, 9:57). Specific areas to which the Act pertains include such activities as:

1. Recruitment, advertising, and application processing;
2. Hiring, upgrading, promotion, tenure, demotion, transfer, layoffs, termination, and rehiring;
3. Rates of pay and other forms of compensation;
4. Job assignments, job classifications, position descriptions, progression, and seniority list;
5. Leave of absence, sick leave, and other leave;
6. Fringe benefits;
7. Selection and financial support for training;
8. Employer sponsored social and recreational programs; and
9. Any other terms or conditions or privileges for the employee (12, 84.111).

In addition, the law imposes on the employer the duty to make reasonable accommodations for the physical or mental impairment of the individual which do not impose an undue hardship on the organization. Reasonable accommodation includes such things as modification of work schedules, job restructuring, and physical modifications relative to the office or job (39, 9:57). Obviously such terms as "undue hardship" and "reasonable accommodation" are open to considerable interpretation, presumably future litigation will assist in clarifying the impact on employers.

An employer is prohibited from asking an applicant about his or her handicap but may ask if the applicant feels capable of performing the job in question. This essentially serves to shift the responsibility of evaluating capabilities from the employer to the prospective employee. Institutions subject to the legislation must submit an assurance of compliance to the U.S. Department of Health and Human Services, and construction programs undertaken by covered institutions must contain provisions that aid access for handicapped persons. Finally, all facilities had until June 8, 1980, to make the necessary modifications to provide reasonable access for the handicapped.

The Rehabilitation Act of 1973 is legislation which should be of particular interest to physical therapists because of their expertise involving handicapped individuals and because this constitutes an area in which they can provide effective consultation.

Summary and Recommendations

Since the mid-1960s, government has occupied an ever increasing role in the employer-employee relationship. The rights of employees have been greatly expanded in an effort to eliminate the discrimination and unfairness which had existed in the past. In addition, the requirements for licensure and accreditation have been strengthened in an effort to ensure that the care provided by the professions and in health care institutions is of the highest quality.

The responsibility of implementing and maintaining the employee rights that are made available by governmental requirements rests primarily on the employer. Physical therapists who occupy managerial and supervisory positions will be directly involved with the types of legislation discussed in this section and must acquire and maintain familiarity with the requirements. The latter (maintaining familiarity) is most important because rules and regulations are constantly being revised.

Past experience indicates that physical therapists advance rather rapidly in the practice of their profession to positions of managerial and supervisory responsibility. Physical therapists who have just entered, or are about to enter, the practice of the profession would be well-advised to start early to develop a working knowledge of the governmental requirements discussed in this section.

References

1. American Law Institute: *Restatement of the Law of Contracts*. American Law Publishers, St. Paul, 1933.
2. American Physical Therapy Association: Standards for Physical Therapy Services, adopted by Board of Directors 1971, adopted by House of Delegates 1975, and amended 1978, 1979, and 1980; and Standards for the Physical Therapy Practitioner, adopted by Board of Directors 1972, adopted by House of Delegates 1975, and amended 1980. American Physical Therapy Association, Washington, 1980.
3. Barber v. Time, Inc., 159 S.W. 2d, 292 (1942).
4. Baxter, E.: Personal communication (In-House Counsel, American Physical Therapy Association, Washington, D.C.)

5. Beth Israel Hospital v. NLRB, 437 U.S. 483 (1978).
6. Blair v. Armour and Co., 306 S.W. 2d, 84 (1957).
7. Byrne v. Boadle, Court of Exchequer of England, 2 H & C 722, 159 Eng. Reports 299 (1863).
8. Darling v. Charleston Memorial Hospital, 33 Ill. 2d. 326, 211 N.E. 2d, 253 (1965).
9. Erickson v. Dilgard, 44 Misc. 2d, 27, 252 N.Y.S. 2d 705 (1962).
10. Fair Labor Standard's Act.
11. 42 United States Code.
12. 45 Code of Federal Regulations.
13. Gadsen General Hospital v. Hamilton, 212 Ala. 351, 103 So. 553 (1923).
14. Gentile v. DeVirgilis, 138 A. 540 (Pa.) (1927).
15. Griggs v. Duke Power Co., 401 U.S., 424 (1971).
16. Health Law Center: *Hospital Law Manual*. Aspen Systems Corporation, Pittsburgh, Vol. II-IIA-IIB, 1974.
17. Heaton v. Ferrell, 325 S.W. 2d, 800 (1959).
18. Herrick v. Wixom, 121 Mich. 384, 80 N.W. 117 (1899).
19. James, C.A., Jr.: Medico-legal considerations in the practice of physical therapy, Phys. Ther. *50:* 1203–1207, 1970.
20. Joint Commission on Accreditation of Hospitals: *Accreditation Manual for Hospitals, 1980.* Joint Commission on Accreditation of Hospitals, Chicago, 1980.
21. Kraff, M. M.: Personal communication (Director of Risk Management, Missouri Professional Liability Insurance Association, Jefferson City, Mo.).
22. Mapp v. Cedars of Lebanon Hospital, Inc., 247 So. 2d, 521 (1971).
23. Missouri Revised Statutes, 1969.
24. Morris, J. A.: *Malpractice Self-Insurance-Alternatives*, Presented, 11th Annual Meeting, American Society of Hospital Attorneys, June 25–26, 1978, San Diego, California-American Hospital Association, Chicago, Illinois, 1978.
25. National Health Lawyers Association: Health Law Update. National Health Lawyers Association, Washington, D.C., 1979.
26. National Labor Relations Act.
27. National League of Cities v. Usery, 426 U. S. 833 (1976).
28. NLRB v. Baptist Hospital, U. S. Supreme Court No. 78-233 (1979).
29. Office of the General Counsel, Memorandum No. 79-76, October 1979.
30. Palsgraf v. Long Island Railroad Co., 248 N.Y. 339, 162 N.E. 99 (1928).
31. Prosser, W. L.: *Handbook of the Law of Torts*, 4th ed. West Publishing Co., St. Paul, 1971.
32. Public Law 95-555.
33. Public Law 95-552.
34. Regan, L. J.: *Doctor, Patient and the Law*, 2nd ed. C. V. Mosby Co., St. Louis, 1949.
35. Rehabilitation Act of 1973.
36. Review Journal of the Federation of American Hospitals, February, Vol. 10, No. 1, 1977.
37. Schumacher, W. A. and Langsdorf, G. F.: *Cyclopedic Law Dictionary*, 3rd ed. Callaghan and Co., Chicago, 1940.
38. Seldon v. City of Sterling, 45 N.E. 2d, 029 (1942).
39. Skolar, M., Abbott, R. and Hays, B.: *Health Care Labor Manual*. Aspen Systems Corporation, Germantown, MD. 1974.
40. Spicer v. Hannah, 247 S.W. 2d., 864 (1952).
41. Thompson v. Otis Elevator Co., 324 S.W. 2d, 755 (1959).
42. Title VII.
43. Trans World Airlines v. Hardeson, 432 U. S. 63 (1977).
44. 29 Code of Federal Regulations.
45. 29 United States Code.
46. U. S. Department of Health, Education, and Welfare: Medical Malpractice Claims. U. S. Department of Health, Education, and Welfare, Washington, 1978.
47. U. S. Department of Labor: Impact of the 1974 Amendment to the National Labor Relations Act. U. S. Department of Labor, Washington, 1979.

chapter 7

FISCAL MANAGEMENT

James B. McKillip

This chapter presents the rationale for, and the basic principles of, fiscal management of a physical therapy service. The examples in the chapter are directed to the physical therapy service in a hospital setting, but the principles apply just as well to any setting including the private office, nursing home, or specialized center.

Examples of cost accounting and budgeting are provided to illustrate the principles of fiscal management. These examples may look laborious and even a bit old-fashioned to the reader familiar with computerized fiscal operations. No apology is offered for the paper-and-pencil examples in this chapter because working through them, as the reader should do, is the most effective way of learning and understanding the elements that go into fiscal management. In that sense, learning how to use fiscal management is similar to learning how to use computerized operations; in both cases, the user must know what to put into the system in order to get something sensible out.

The examples contain items, categories, and formulas that may vary slightly from setting to setting. The principles, however, are fairly uniform across a wide variety of clinical settings and even in academic and business settings.

GENERAL STATEMENTS

Definition and Perspective

Fiscal management is the method of controlling the economics of problems at hand. Specifically, for the purpose of this chapter, it is an activity concerned with discovering, developing, defining, and evaluating financial goals of the physical therapy department. Such an activity is usually assumed to be the responsibility of administrators or managers. Yet the success of this activity is many times dependent upon the combined efforts of all levels of the staff of an organization. Some authorities prefer the term business administration to fiscal management because they feel that business administration connotes less rigid control than fiscal management, and that fiscal management is only a part of business administration. Whatever the phraseology preferred, the end result should be sagacious evaluation and implementation of all the goals the department is trying to achieve. It is only after gathering all the facts, analyzing them, and understanding how these facts interact with all of the other components of a problem that cogent management decisions can be made.

Sound fiscal management is essential to the ongoing success of providing physical therapy services. As essential as it is to be financially secure, such security is not the main nor even the secondary goal of the physical therapy department. The primary goal is usually service to the patient. When the economics of health care come first, there usually follow deficits in quality, quantity, and the effectiveness of the care. If sound financial management is in its proper perspective, it can do much to augment the quality, quantity, and effectiveness of health care by providing a system that makes the service available and accessible at a reasonable cost.

Components

A system for discovering, developing, defining, and evaluating the costs of a physical therapy department should also have as a by-product the identification of all components necessary to provide the service. Such identification can also lead to a thorough understanding of all of those components. In physical therapy, the general components of service are labor, equipment, and overhead applied over time. Each of these components has specific facets which, when documented and extrapolated, provide greater understanding of the component. Such specifics can be used as pieces of a jigsaw puzzle to define or identify the service. These specifics can also be used to help evaluate the service as well as to project needs and develop budgets. For instance, to develop a personnel budget one must know the volume of the patient load, the character of that patient load, the kind of space available for the treatment to be rendered in, and the kind and amount of equipment needed, to name just a few of the necessary specifics. The details of such specifics, as well as others, will all interact with and affect each other. When these details are identified because of fiscal concern, the by-product of their identification can be more intelligent planning, developing, and analysis of the service. Regardless of the size or location of the department, it is necessary to understand and to solve problems of recruiting, managing, and training personnel; establishing salary scales and fringe benefits; scheduling physical therapists and patients; planning budgets; purchasing equipment and supplies; establishing fee schedules; determining methods for billing; handling accounts receivable; integrating the physical therapy service with other services of the health facility; and participating in public relations programs. Once acquainted with problems such as these, one must have a way to evaluate and control them. Financial management provides, either directly or indirectly, a realistic look at all of the aspects of the physical therapy department. Table 7.1 diagrammatically outlines the components that could

Table 7.1

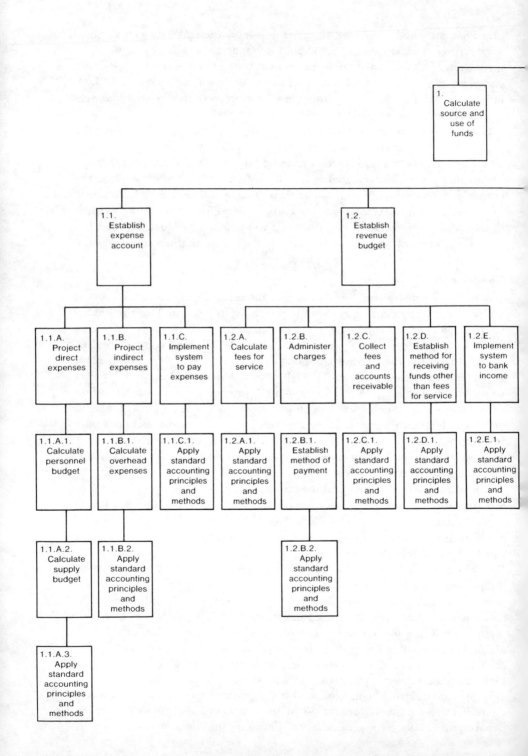

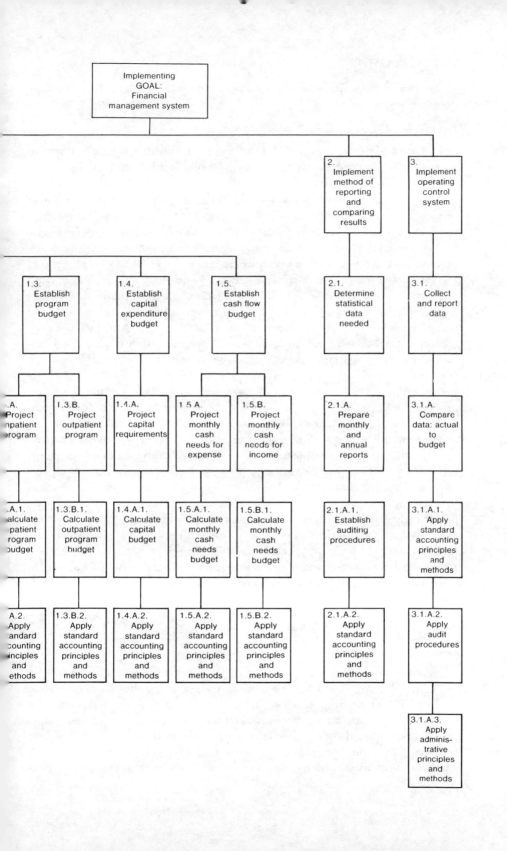

Implementing
GOAL:
Financial
management system

2.
Implement
method of
reporting
and
comparing
results

3.
Implement
operating
control
system

1.3.
Establish
program
budget

1.4.
Establish
capital
expenditure
budget

1.5.
Establish
cash flow
budget

2.1.
Determine
statistical
data
needed

3.1.
Collect
and report
data

.A.
Project
inpatient
program

1.3.B.
Project
outpatient
program

1.4.A.
Project
capital
requirements

1.5.A.
Project
monthly
cash
needs for
expense

1.5.B.
Project
monthly
cash
needs for
income

2.1.A.
Prepare
monthly
and
annual
reports

3.1.A.
Compare
data: actual
to
budget

.A.1.
Calculate
inpatient
program
budget

1.3.B.1.
Calculate
outpatient
program
budget

1.4.A.1.
Calculate
capital
budget

1.5.A.1.
Calculate
monthly
cash
needs
budget

1.5.B.1.
Calculate
monthly
cash
needs
budget

2.1.A.1.
Establish
auditing
procedures

3.1.A.1.
Apply
standard
accounting
principles
and
methods

.A.2.
Apply
standard
accounting
principles
and
methods

1.3.B.2.
Apply
standard
accounting
principles
and
methods

1.4.A.2.
Apply
standard
accounting
principles
and
methods

1.5.A.2.
Apply
standard
accounting
principles
and
methods

1.5.B.2.
Apply
standard
accounting
principles
and
methods

2.1.A.2.
Apply
standard
accounting
principles
and
methods

3.1.A.2.
Apply
audit
procedures

3.1.A.3.
Apply
adminis-
trative
principles
and
methods

be used in implementing a fiscal management system for a physical therapy department.

Necessary Skills and Knowledge

The price of success as a physical therapy administrator is the effort needed to acquire skills and knowledge that are only incidentally related to the profession of physical therapy. These skills and knowledge bring an awareness to the physical therapy administrator that there is more to a professional service than mastering and using physical therapy techniques. The knowledge necessary for fiscal management includes an understanding of applied logic and mathematics, summary data and statistics, accounting, systems development and analysis, economics, business administration, and organization theory. In the main, one learns the skills and knowledge by guided or trial-and-error experiences, through in-service education from the health facility administrative personnel, through continuing education or instructional courses provided by the American Physical Therapy Association or its components, through formal education, or, as most do, through a combination of the preceding. Generally, the more complex the setting within which the professional works, the more the problems and responsibilities and the greater the need for sound fiscal management. It is also true that the secret of a busy, successful, one-person physical therapy department is good organization and management of that therapist's time, skills, and resources. Regardless of the size or complexity of the physical therapy department, the physical therapist responsible for managing or administering the department should certainly have a voice in establishing and controlling the fiscal aspects of providing and charging for the service delivered to patients. The physical therapist administrator of a bigger or more complex, or more comprehensive, physical therapy department will require considerable skills and knowledge as a physical therapy professional and as a business person. The wage and benefit package for the physical therapist manager or administrator should reflect the complexity of responsibilities and the required skills and knowledge and should be commensurate with comparable positions in the professional and business world.

COST ACCOUNTING

Definition

Generally, cost accounting includes the theories, methods, and procedures for identifying, accumulating, measuring, and reporting the cost of obtaining or providing something specific. In cost accounting, every item must be identified, and a dollar value established for it. It makes no difference how an item is acquired—gift, grant, purchase with hard cash, or purchase on credit; a value must be established for it and that value must be counted. There are probably as many cost accounting formulas as there are accountants. The health facility's comptroller can give the appropriate information about the formulas used in a particular facility. Because these formulas are usually more involved than budgets, it is imperative to discuss them with the comptroller to appreciate the how and why of various cost allocations. Actually, some parts of these formulas can be, and are, used in establishing departmental budgets.

Chart of Accounts

For any accounting system to be effective, it must have the necessary components and organization to accurately accumulate, communicate, and interpret historical, current, and projected quantitative data relating to a specific activity (2).

A basic accounting method for organizing data is referred to as a chart of accounts. The chart of accounts for individual health facilities may differ, dependent upon the facility's size and complexity. Differences may also be found in the chart of accounts for the various components within an entity. The chart should be designed to allow for contraction and expansion to meet specific requirements of a component or an adjustment of goals and yet maintain a basic uniformity for recording and reporting financial information.

Most charts of accounts are number coded for ease of identification and organization, and for the processing of activity related to the system. An example of a basic chart of accounts and an overall numbering system is shown in Table 7.2. Further information on this topic, not essential to the purpose of this chapter, can be found in AHA's publication "Chart of Accounts for Hospitals" (2).

Budgets

Budgets are educated estimates of future needs within a specific time frame, based upon past records, personal experience, knowledge, and projected planning (1). A master budget contains all the budgets of all departments in a facility. These usually include the operational, capital and cash flow budgets. The operational budget usually includes the expense, income, and program budgets. The capital budget is calculated separately, and the cash flow budget incorporates the operational and capital budgets. The facility must have certain essential organizational characteristics before budgets can be effective in financial planning:

1. An organizational structure with responsibilities specifically defined and assigned;
2. An accounting system and procedure paralleling the departmental organization of the facility;
3. The participation of responsible personnel at all levels of management in budget preparation;

Table 7.2
Chart of Accounts

110–196 Assets	
110–114	Operating fund
120–122	Specific purpose fund
130–132	Endowment fund
140–146	Plant fund
150–155	Construction fund
160–196	Other funds
217–298 Liabilities	
217	Operating fund
227	Specific purpose fund
237–238	Endowment fund
247–248	Plant fund
257–258	Construction fund
267–298	Other funds
219–299 Capital Accounts	
219	Operating fund
229	Specific purpose fund
239	Endowment fund
249	Plant fund
259	Construction fund
310–599 Revenue Accounts	
310–499	Patient service revenue
500–529	Deductions from revenue
530–599	Other revenue
600–999 Expense Accounts	
600–699	Nursing service
700–799	Other professional services
800–899	General services
900–949	Fiscal services
950–979	Administrative services
980–999	Unassigned expenses

4. An understanding by all those involved in budget preparation of the service ideals of the facility as well as its financial goals; and
5. An adequate reporting system that provides historical and current reliable financial and statistical information to personnel responsible for budget preparation (1).

Budgets can be established for all the various needs of a physical therapy department—personnel, equipment, expendable supplies, cash flow, and so forth. The comptroller, or his equivalent, in a health facility can acquaint the responsible physical therapist with the manner in which the facility wants budgets submitted, and can assist the physical therapy administrator in understanding and establishing the department's budgets. It is also important for the physical therapy administrator to understand how the physical therapy budget must conform to the total budget and goals of the health facility.

Budgets can be rigid, but in most instances they should be flexible enough to allow one to work successfully toward established goals. Budgets should be based on a primary study of the goals of the physical therapy department and the health facility. After a budget has been reviewed and the facts are coldly visible, it may be necessary to adjust the objectives and the budget. Such adjustments permit a more realistic approach to the function of budgets.

Expenses

There are two major classes of expenses: direct and indirect. Direct expenses are those that are directly incurred by the physical therapy department, such as salaries and supplies. Equipment purchases are usually considered not as direct expenses but as capital expenditures in a capital budget. Indirect expenses are those incurred by the facility as a whole to support all departments and shared, by allocation, in the expense budgets of all departments including physical therapy. Indirect expenses include such things as employee benefits, laundry, housekeeping, equipment depreciation, plant operation and maintenance, and administration. Employee benefits include all those nonsalary and nonwage costs that the facility must bear when it hires employees. These include the costs of all fringe benefits such as vacation, insurance (malpractice, health, and accident), sick leave, continuing education, attendance at professional meetings, uniforms and laundry, and any other benefits that might be provided for employees by the facility at the facility's cost.

Expenses can also be described as fixed or variable. An example of a fixed indirect expense would be rent. Rent will remain the same no matter how many treatments are provided in the given space. An example of a variable indirect expense would be the laundry expense. The laundry costs will increase or decrease dependent upon how much linen is used on how many patients. Knowing which expenses are fixed and which are variable will help to identify the impact these expenses will have upon the costs of the physical therapy service.

Income

After all costs have been established to meet the needs of current operations, expansion of physical plant, education, research, and anything else that costs money, provision to meet these costs must be made. These goals can usually be accomplished by generating income or revenue (1, 2). Income can be in one or any combination of forms: fees, grants or donations of money, equipment, or time. To continue to provide the service, the income must at least meet expenses. That is, somehow someone must pay for expenses of the service. An income budget is a primary part of any facility's overall budget.

Most health facilities hope that their physical therapy departments will make a profit to support or provide other services within a health facility, or to provide incentive for their professionals' efforts and investments. If there is to be profit, there must also be some formula to calculate how much the profit should be.

Application of Cost Accounting

Once a physical therapy administrator is familiar with the principles of cost accounting, he can apply these principles to study all facets of the department and to assist in making administrative decisions. Cost accounting provides a hard, cold, realistic financial look at what it costs to provide the service. Physical therapists deal in medical services, so their approach cannot always be cold, hard, and financially rigid. A good physical therapy administrator will use the information gained from budgeting and cost accounting to best service the facility, its patients, and staff (12).

One important use of cost accounting principles and methods is in preparation of an operating budget.

Table 7.3
Projected Operating Budget* Physical Therapy Department any Hospital 1981

Revenue		
Projected number of treatments		
(based on 1980 plus a 5 percent projected growth factor for 1981):	17,000	
Average fee per treatment:	$ 24.50	
Gross revenue	17,000 × 24.50 =	$416,500
Deductions and allowances[a]		41,650
Net revenue		374,850
Direct expenses		
1. Salaries and wages[b, c]	177,672	
2. Supplies[a]	3,000	
Total Direct Expenses		180,672
Indirect expenses		
1. Employee benefits[b, c]	42,252	
2. Equipment depreciation	10,000	
3. Building and land improvements and leasehold improvement: Depreciation and rent	10,227	
4. Operation of the plant[a]	13,488	
5. Maintenance of the plant[a]	13,000	
6. Housekeeping[a]	8,200	
7. Laundry and Linen[a]	4,400	
8. Administration[a]	48,000	
Total Indirect Expenses		149,567
Total Expenses		330,239
Net Operating Revenue (Net revenue less total expenses)		$ 44,611

* Annualized, using actual data from the first six months of 1980.

[a] Reflects a projected 10 percent increase of these expenses as annualized using first six months of 1980.

[b] Reflects a cost of living increase of nine percent.

[c] Reflects a projected increased cost for more professional labor in servicing a projected five percent increase in the patient load.

PROJECTED OPERATING BUDGET

This section of the chapter presents step-by-step details on the cost accounting methods that can be used in preparation of a projected operating budget. The steps and formulas presented come from several sources (1, 2, 7, 11). While the details of these steps and formulas may vary slightly from facility to facility—dependent upon methods used by the particular facility's comptroller—the principles of using such steps and formulas vary little if at all.

For the worked examples that are presented, assume throughout a physical therapy department in a short-term, acute care facility, with five full-time physical therapists, one full-time physical therapist assistant, two full-time physical therapy aides, one full-time secretary-clerk, and the necessary part-time and temporary personnel to help provide services on weekends and during holidays. Further assumptions about space, the facility's total direct expenses, and so forth are given when appropriate.

Table 7.3 presents the projected operating budget for this physical therapy department. This table would ordinarily be the *final* step in the process, but it is presented first here so that the reader can see the end product and relate it to the methods that follow. The reader who is unfamiliar with budgets should, before studying the detailed methods, examine Table 7.3 closely and double-check the arithmetic to get a full appreciation of the terms "gross," "net," "direct," "indirect," and "total."

The details that follow focus on the calculation of direct expenses and indirect expenses. The calculation of gross revenue shown in Table 7.3 is based on certain considerations about productivity and scheduling of fees, two topics which are discussed in the next section on Other Uses of Cost Accounting.

Direct Expenses

Salaries and Wages

Table 7.3 projects a total figure of $177,672 for all of the department's salaries and wages. This figure includes salaries and wages only; it does not include payroll taxes, insurance, leave, and other costs that are classified as personnel benefits under indirect expenses. Column 2 in Table 7.4, Projected Monthly Payroll Costs, projects the monthly salaries and wages for all full-time, part-time, and temporary employees in the department. The reader should satisfy himself that the total salaries and wages figure of $177,672 in Table 7.3 represents 12 times the monthly total of $14,806 shown in column 2, Table 7.4.

The first column in Table 7.4 shows the department's various employee positions. The assumption was made that two part-time physical therapists and one part-time physical therapy aide would be needed to augment the full-time staff in providing weekend physical therapy services. Another assumption was that four temporary physical therapists and one temporary aide would be needed to provide services for six hours on each of nine

Table 7.4
Projected Monthly Payroll Costs*

1	2	3	4	5	6	7	8	9	10	11	12	13	14	15	16	17	18
			Employee Benefits														
Staff	Salaries and Wages	Payroll Taxes	Malprac-tice and Li-ability In-surance	H.A.M.M. Insurance	Group Life Insur-ance	Group Disa-bility Insur-ance	Group Pension Plan	Vaca-tion	Holi-days	Educa-tion Leave	Sick Leave	Uni-forms	Total Em-ployee Benefits	Total Payroll Cost	Maxi-mum Hours Worked and Paid	Maxi-mum Avail-able Hours Patient Treat-ment	Maxi-mum Potential Patient Treat-ment
Director	2295	132	14	32	6	20	92	159	29	119	53	10	666	2961	174	—	—
Supervisor	2066	127	14	32	4	18	83	123	36	62	48	10	557	2623	174	86	198
Staff Part-time (PT)																	
1	1600	98	14	32	2	14	64	123		31	36	10	424	2024	174	174	405
2	1530	94	14	32	2	13	61	123		31	35	10	415	1945	174	174	405
3	1411	86	14	32	2	12	56	92		31	33	10	368	1779	174	174	405
P.T.Assistant	1148	70	14	32	2	10	46	66		22	26	10	296	1444	174	174	405
Aides																	
1	780	48	8	32	2	7	31	45		6	18	10	207	987	174		
2	780	48	8	32	2	7	31	45		6	18	10	207	987	174		
Secretary-Clerk	1000	61	8	32	2	9	40	58		4	23	10	247	1247	174		
Weekend (PT):																	
PT $86 × 9 Days	774	47											47	821	63	63	160
PT $86 × 9 Days	774	47											47	821	63	63	160
Aide $40 × 9 Days	360	22											22	382	63	—	—
Holidays (PT):																	
PT $86 × 9 Days/12 mo																	
PT $86 × 9 Days/12 mo																	
PT $86 × 9 Days/12 mo																	
PT $86 × 9 Days/12 mo																	
Aide $40 × 9 Days/12mo																	
Average monthly cost	288	18											18	306	23	18	42
Totals	14806	898	108	288	24	110	504	834	65	312	290	90	3521	18327	1778	926	2180

holidays through the year, the number of holidays observed by the facility in this example. Column 2 in Table 7.4 projects the average monthly wages of these temporary employees.

Supplies

The projected direct expense of $3,000 for supplies covers anticipated purchases of consumable supplies and equipment items that generally cost less than $100 each. For this example, the estimate of $3,000 came from the author's own experience. The estimate should take into account the experience of the previous year, anticipated growth in number of treatments and personnel, anticipated changes in types of patients seen, and inflationary trends in prices.

Indirect Expenses

Employee Benefits

Table 7.3 projects an indirect expense of $42,252 for employee benefits in the department's budget. This expense is usually allocated to the department as a proportion of the facility's total expense for employee benefits. The percentage used in making the allocation is taken from the ratio of:

$$\frac{\text{Department's direct expense for salaries and wages}}{\text{Facility's direct expense for salaries and wages}}.$$

From Table 7.3, the department's projected salaries and wages amount to $177,672 (or $14,806 monthly in Table 7.4, column 2). Assume that the facility's projected salaries and wages amount to $3,553,440 (or $296,120 per month). Then,

$$\frac{177,672}{3,553,440} \quad \text{or} \quad \frac{14,806}{296,120} = 0.05 \quad \text{or} \quad 5 \text{ percent.}$$

Assuming that the facility's total expense for employee benefits is projected to be $845,040 (or $70,420 per month), the department's allocation of indirect expense for employee benefits will be 5 percent of the facility's expense for employee benefits or $42,252 ($3,521 monthly).

The method just shown for calculating the department's allocation of employee benefits as an indirect expense illustrates two important cost-accounting principles in projecting indirect expenses.

1. Expenses incurred by the facility as a whole and not directly attributable to, or subject to the control of, any one department must be allocated on a proportional basis to all departments; in fact, this proportional allocation defines indirect expenses.
2. The proportional allocation of a facility expense as an indirect expense to the various departments is usually based on a factor reasonably related to the size of the expense to be allocated (in the example, the size of the facility's expense for employee benefits is related to the size

of the expense for salaries and wages; as a general rule, the employee benefits package of a facility adds an expense equal to anywhere from 21 to 35 percent of the salaries and wages—in the example, the additional expense is 23.8 percent).

One more point about the allocation of an indirect expense should be made here: The factor used in determining the proportional allocation of an indirect expense to one department is also used in determining the proportional allocations of that same indirect expense to all other departments—only the percentages will vary. The point is a good one to keep in mind in case you ever seek a change in the basis on which an indirect expense is allocated to your department. You would have to seek a change in the basis or general rule for all departments, not just your own.

Table 7.4 offers another, more detailed, cost accounting view of employee benefits projected for the example physical therapy department. Columns 3 through 13 (Payroll Taxes through Uniforms) in Table 7.4 present each employee benefit, the projected cost of each benefit for each employee, and the projected total cost of each benefit. Column 14 (Total Employee Benefits) summarizes all of these figures.

Several things should be noted about columns 3 through 14 in Table 7.4 before considering where the detailed figures came from. First, payroll taxes are usually included, by most accountants, in the category of employee benefits—the full title of the category should be "payroll taxes and employee benefits" but this chapter adheres to customary practice. Second, notice that payroll taxes apply to all personnel, and that employee benefits (in the true sense of the word) apply only to full-time personnel. These applications are typical. Now, notice the total monthly cost projected for all employee benefits. The total of $3,521 at the foot of column 14 represents ¹⁄₁₂ of the $42,252 projected for the department's employee benefits in Table 7.3. Various budgets, prepared for different purposes, should "add up" or be consistent in this way.

The following information describes how the detailed figures were obtained for columns 3 through 13 in Table 7.4. The dollar figures in the worked examples shown below have been rounded to the nearest dollar in Table 7.4. In some of the examples, the reader will notice the use of "173.33 hours" as a divisor—that figure represents the maximum number of hours worked and paid each month for each full-time employee (see column 16 in Table 7.4, where the figure is rounded to 174). More will be said about that figure, and columns 16 through 18 in Table 7.4, in the subsequent section of this chapter.

Column 3, Payroll Taxes. Payroll taxes in 1980 were 6.13 percent (6.13 percent paid by the employer and 6.13 percent paid by the employee on the first $25,900 of gross earned income). The director of the department is the only employee who will earn more than $25,900 in the example department ($2,295 × 12 = $27,540). The monthly payroll tax incurred by the facility and allocated to the department for that position is:

$$(\$25,900 \times .0613 = \$1587.67)/12 = \$132.31.$$

For all other employees, the payroll tax rate is applied directly to the monthly salary, for example:

$$\$2,066 \times .0613 = \$126.65$$
$$\$1,600 \times .0613 = 98.08$$

Column 4, Malpractice and Liability Insurance. Assuming that the physical therapy service in the example is a contracted service, premiums were calculated for a contracted service from the 1980 rates of Maginnis and Associates for $1,000,000 of malpractice liability coverage. The monthly cost of this insurance for each employee, as shown in Table 7.4, consist of two parts—a charge for the service and a charge for the individual. The annual premium charge for the service includes $246 for the contractor, $65 for general liability, $65 for non-auto liability, $32 personal liability, and $32 for the facility as an additional insured, or $440 total, or $440/9 employees = $48.88 per employee. For each physical therapist and each physical therapist assistant, there are additional annual premium charges of $36 as an employee and $82 as a therapist or assistant, or a total of $48.88 + 36 + 82 = $166.80, or a monthly cost of $166.80/12 = $13.90. For each aide and the secretary-clerk, the additional annual premium charges are $13 as an employee and $29 as an aide or other, or a total of $48.88 + 13 + 29 = $90.88, or a monthly cost of $90.88/12 = $7.57.

Column 5, Health, Accident, and Major Medical Group Insurance (H.A.M.M.). The monthly premium rate for each employee is $32.06.

Column 6, Group Life Insurance. The monthly premium rate is $0.42 for each $1,000 of insurance. The director has $15,000 of insurance ($0.42 × 15 = $6.30), the supervisor $10,000, and each remaining employee $5,000.

Column 7, Group Disability Insurance. The monthly premium rate is $0.0087 per dollar of gross monthly salary. For the director, $0.0087 × $2,295 = $19.97.

Column 8, Group Pension Plan. The monthly contribution is 1 percent of the gross monthly salary. For the director, .04 × $2,295 = $91.80.

Column 9, Vacation. Vacation costs are calculated at the rate of the replacement who assumes the job responsibilities of the vacationer. For the director, the replacement is the supervisor; for the supervisor, it is the top of the staff; and for each of the rest of the physical therapists on the staff, it is the physical therapy staff relief calculated at a rate of $1,600 per month. For all others, the assumption is that vacation relief can be secured at the rate of their monthly salary equivalents. Vacation for the director is 20 days, for the supervisor 20 days, for two physical therapists 20 days each, for one physical therapist 15 days, and for all others 15 days each. The computation of the prorated monthly vacation cost for the director uses the monthly salary of the supervisor for determining the annual cost of 20 days vacation replacement. This annual cost is then prorated over 12 months. The computation is as follows:

1. Cost/hour: $\dfrac{\$2,066/\text{month}}{173.33 \text{ hours/month}} = \$11.92/\text{hour}$
2. Cost/day: $\$11.92/\text{hour} \times 8 \text{ hours} = \$95.36/\text{day}$
3. Cost/year: $\$95.36/\text{day} \times 20 \text{ days} = \$1,907.20/\text{year}$
4. Cost/month: $\$1,907.20/12 = \$158.93/\text{month}$

Column 10, Holidays. Notice, first, that columns 2 and 3 in Table 7.4 show the costs in wages and payroll taxes for temporary personnel to provide holiday coverage. Column 10 shows the cost of having the director and supervisor alternate duty for holidays at the same rate as the temporary physical therapists, namely $86 per holiday. The director works four holidays, the supervisor five. The prorated monthly cost for the director is:

$$(\$86 \times 4 \text{ days} = \$344/\text{year})/12 = \$28.67,$$

and this is entered in column 10 as $29.

Column 11, Educational Leave. Educational leave costs are calculated at the rate of the replacement who assumes the job responsibilities of the person on educational leave. See the succession of replacement described for column 9, Vacation, above. Educational leave for the director is 15 days, for the supervisor 10 days, for the other physical therapists and the physical therapist assistant 5 days each, for the aides 2 days each, and for the secretary-clerk 1 day. The computation of the prorated monthly educational leave cost for the director uses the monthly salary of the supervisor to determine the annual cost of 15 days educational leave replacement, then this annual cost is prorated over 12 months. The computation is as follows:

1. Cost/hour: $\dfrac{\$2,066/\text{month}}{173.33 \text{ hours/month}} = \$11.92/\text{hour}$
2. Cost/day: $\$11.92/\text{hour} \times 8 \text{ hours} = \$95.36/\text{day}$
3. Cost/year: $\$95.36/\text{day} \times 15 \text{ days} = \$1,430.40/\text{year}$
4. Cost/month: $\$1,430.40/12 = \$119.20/\text{month}$

Column 12, Sick Leave. Each employee is entitled to 12 sick leave days per year. Assuming that each employee will use 4 sick leave days, and will be paid 1 day for every 4 days of the remaining unused 8 sick leave days, and assuming that part-time personnel will be called in to work for the person on sick leave, the calculation of sick leave costs is based on 6 days per year prorated over 12 months. The calculation of the prorated monthly sick leave cost for the director is as follows:

1. Cost/hour: $\dfrac{\$2,295/\text{month}}{173.33 \text{ hours/month}} = \$13.24/\text{hour}$
2. Cost/day: $\$13.24/\text{hour} \times 8 \text{ hours} = \$105.92/\text{day}$
3. Cost/year: $\$105.92/\text{day} \times 6 \text{ days} = \$635.52 \text{ year}$
4. Cost/month: $\$635.52/12 = \$52.96/\text{month}.$

Column 13, Uniforms. Each employee is entitled to have one uniform laundered every other working day. Given 22 working days per month, the laundering of 11 uniforms per month at a cost of $.90 per uniform amounts to $9.90 per month per employee.

Finally, on the topic of employee benefits, the reader should now appreciate that the costs to the facility—ultimately to the department—of seven of the eleven personnel benefits are directly related to the direct expense of salaries and wages. The interested reader can, in fact, add the totals of columns 3, 7, 8, 9, 10, 11, and 12 in Table 7.4 and find that the total monthly cost of these seven benefits represents *86 percent* of the total monthly cost for all benefits (see column 14, Table 7.4). The method presented earlier for allocating personnel benefits as an indirect expense to the department, on the basis of the department's proportional direct expense for salaries and wages, appears to be quite reasonable.

Equipment Depreciation

The figure of $10,000 shown for equipment depreciation in Table 7.3, the Projected Operating Budget, is an estimate based on the author's experience. If the example were not hypothetical, the following principles and instructions would apply.

To project the department's annual equipment depreciation, set up a depreciation schedule on each item of professional and office equipment (usually limited to items costing over $100). Establish the expected useful life (in years) of each item. Determine the annual depreciation of each item by dividing the expected useful life into the cost. As an example, the annual depreciation of an ultrasound device, purchased at $1,600 and with an expected useful life of five years would be:

$$\frac{\$1,600 \text{ cost}}{5 \text{ years}} = \$320.$$

Add the annual depreciations of all items of equipment on the depreciation schedule to obtain the equipment depreciation figure for the projected operating budget.

Purchases of equipment and furnishings costing more than $100 each would not appear in the projected operating budget. Such purchases would appear in a capital budget. The Projected Capital Budget for the example physical therapy department is presented in Table 7.5. Notice that the totals in Table 7.5 do not appear in Table 7.3, but realize that the annual depreciations of the equipment items would be included in the equipment depreciation figure in Table 7.3.

Building and Land Improvements and Leasehold Improvement: Depreciation and Rent

The title of this category of indirect expense is a complicated description of "rent." The indirect expense for the physical therapy department is determined as a percentage of the facility's total cost for "rent." The

Table 7.5
Projected Capital Budget Physical Therapy Department any Hospital 1981

Professional equipment			
1. 1 set electronically adjustable parallel bars		$4500.00	
2. 3 intermittent traction machines	@ $1722.00	5166.00	
3. 2 electronically adjustable tables	@ $2963.00	5926.00	
4. 2 tens units	@ $ 318.00	636.00	
5. 1 bicycle ergonometer		901.00	
6. 1 adjustable treadmill		2836.00	
Total professional equipment			$19,965.00
Office Equipment			
1. 1 desk		450.00	
2. 1 chair		95.00	
3. 1 electronic printing calculator		165.00	
4. 1 IBM typewriter		2300.00	
5. 1 dictaphone transcriber		1450.00	
Total office equipment			$ 4,460.00
Total professional and office equipment			$24,425.00

percentage applied represents the department's total area in square feet as a proportion of the facility's total area in square feet. Assume, for example, that the facility's total cost for "rent" is $204,540 per year, that the facility's total area is 60,000 square feet, and that the physical therapy department occupies 3,000 square feet of the facility's space. Calculation of the department's indirect expense for "rent" would then be:

$$\frac{3,000 \text{ square feet}}{60,000 \text{ square feet}} = .05$$

$$\text{and} \quad \$204,540 \times .05 = \$10,227$$

Operation of the Plant

This indirect expense is calculated on the same basis as that described for "rent" immediately above. Assume that the facility's projected cost for operation of the plant is $269,760. The calculation would be:

$$\frac{3,000 \text{ square feet}}{60,000 \text{ square feet}} = .05$$

$$\text{and} \quad \$269,760 \times .05 = \$13,488$$

Maintenance of the Plant

As in the two examples immediately above, this indirect expense is calculated on the basis of proportional area. Assuming a projected facility cost for maintenance of $260,000, the physical therapy department's share would be:

$$\frac{3{,}000 \text{ square feet}}{60{,}000 \text{ square feet}} = .05$$

and $260,000 × .05 = $13,000.

Housekeeping

The figure of $8,200 in Table 7.3 is an estimate based on the author's experience. In the nonhypothetical situation, this figure would be obtained by determining the department's housekeeping time as a percentage of the facility's total housekeeping time (all in person hours), and then applying that percentage to the facility's total projected housekeeping cost.

Laundry and Linen

Again, the figure of $4,400 is an estimate based on experience. This figure would be obtained by determining the physical therapy department's total number of pounds of laundry used as a percentage of the facility's total number of pounds of laundry used, and then applying that percentage to the facility's total projected laundry and linen cost.

Administration

The reader will have noticed that the indirect expense in this category ($48,000; see Table 7.3) is large; in fact, for the hypothetical physical therapy department, this indirect expense is larger than any other indirect expense. A common practice in most institutions and organizations is one of spreading or allocating administration costs among the departments, services, or units of the institution or organization as an indirect expense (or as indirect expenses separated into two or more categories). The recipients of this allocation do not always accept it, or the basis for determining it, with grace.

Consider, first, the kinds of things that make up administration costs: salaries and employee benefits for administrative personnel; all business operations of the facility; insurance (several kinds, including public liability); taxes and licenses; interest and financing expenses; legal fees; and telephone, postage, and so forth. For the most part, these costs are incurred by the very existence of the facility as an entity that includes and is greater than the sum of all of its parts (departments).

Consider, also, that administration activities and costs grow larger as the activities and costs grow larger in the facility's departments. It should come as no surprise, then, that the allocation of administration costs as an indirect expense is based on the proportional size of the department's total direct expenses.

Assume that the facility's total projected direct expenses are $7,106,880 (the sum of all direct expenses from projected operating budgets throughout the facility), and that the facility's total projected administration cost is $1,920,000. Table 7.3 shows that the total direct expenses projected for the physical therapy department are $180,672. The calculation of the department's administration indirect expense is determined proportionally by:

$$\frac{\$\ 180,672}{\$7,106,880} = .025$$

and $\$1,920,000 \times .025 = \$48,000.$

This section of the chapter has presented in considerable detail the cost accounting principles and methods used in preparing a projected operating budget. To emphasize again, the methods and formulas may vary somewhat from facility to facility but the principles are fairly uniform. For example—and now the example will make sense—the various kinds of costs allocated as indirect expenses to the physical therapy department will be allocated no matter what the particular categories, methods, and formulas are. The physical therapist administrator should find out from the facility's comptroller what the categories are and what is included in them, as well as what the methods and formulas are that determine the allocations. Finally, the total direct and indirect expenses of the department's operating budget do give the most accurate and realistic picture of the cost of providing the services of the physical therapy department.

An expression often heard in the corporate world, and more and more in the health care world, is: 'It's the bottom line that counts." The bottom line in table 7.3 shows a net operating revenue (excess of revenue over expense) of $44,611 for the hypothetical physical therapy department. This bottom line depends not just on the cost of providing the service, as was emphasized in this section, but on other considerations such as productivity and fee schedules. Cost accounting can help in these other considerations.

OTHER USES OF COST ACCOUNTING

Once the cost accounting procedures identify, measure, and account for the specific components of providing the physical therapy service, the physical therapist administrator can analyze the data. Each specific component can be studied to see if it is necessary, why it is necessary, what it costs, and if the cost is reasonable. This evaluation can include comparisons with similar departments in the same geographic area. Evaluation of this kind can also lead to a better understanding of what each component in the service or program does and how it interacts with other components.

The cost accounting approach to evaluating the physical therapy service can be especially useful in identifying the necessary actions to effect wiser use of resources and in strengthening the rationale for increased expenditures. This approach can also be used to examine productivity in a variety of ways, to establish the cost per modality or procedure and the cost per patient treatment, and to establish fee schedules.

Productivity

Patient treatment (including evaluation) is the reason for existence of a physical therapy department, and the chief function of the department's personnel is to provide that patient treatment. Not all of the personnel time and cost, however, is committed to this function. In other words, not all of the hours worked and paid for in the department are "productive hours" in terms of treating patients and producing revenue.

Column 16 in Table 7.4 shows the maximum monthly hours worked and paid, as projected for the example physical therapy department. The 174 hours for each full-time employee represents the average monthly hours (rounded up from 173.33 hours) based on 52 40-hour weeks in the year. Column 17 shows the maximum monthly hours available for treating patients. The assumption here is that the director is not available for patient treatment, that the supervisor is only available 50 percent of the time for patient treatment, and that among all of the remaining personnel only the physical therapists and the physical therapist assistant are available (accountable) for patient treatment. A comparison of the total hours in columns 16 and 17 shows that the maximum available hours for patient treatment represent only 52 percent of the maximum hours worked and paid. Not all of the maximum available hours, however, are "productive hours."

In 1955, Rodriquez and Rodriquez stated that the physical therapist's maximum potential treatment productivity should be adjusted down from 100 percent to 70 to 80 percent, because of various downtime factors (15). In the 25 years since 1955, the advance of the team concept, and complexity of professional responsibility to the health facility, the profusion of paper work demanded by third party payers, particularly the federal and state governments, and more involvement with administrative detail have forced the physical therapist to spend more and more time away from treating patients. Today, 65 percent of maximum treatment potential is much more realistic than 80 percent. In many facilities, 60 percent maximum potential would be more realistic.

Going back to the total number of maximum available hours for patient treatment in column 17, Table 7.4, the total expected "productive hours" becomes:

$$926 \text{ hours} \times .65 = 602 \text{ hours/month.}$$

This estimate of productive hours can be useful to the physical therapy administrator in examining productivity from several perspectives. For example:

1. Productive hours as a percentage of maximum hours worked and paid

$$\frac{602 \text{ hours}}{1{,}778 \text{ hours (column 16, Table 7.4)}} = 0.34 \text{ or } 34 \text{ percent.}$$

2. Labor cost per productive hour

$$\frac{\$18,327 \text{ (column 15, Table 7.4)}}{602 \text{ hours}} = \$30.44/\text{productive hour.}$$

Column 18 in Table 7.4 provides a further look at productivity, namely, maximum potential patient treatments that can be carried out within the maximum available hours for patient treatment (column 17). A patient treatment is defined as all care rendered to a patient during any one visit. The figures in column 18 were obtained by calculations for which the following assumptions were made about the number of patient treatments per hour: supervisor 2.30, each full-time staff physical therapist 2.33, each part-time (week-end) physical therapist 2.54, and each temporary (holiday) physical therapist 2.33.

Just as the total maximum hours available for patient treatment (926 hours) was adjusted for various downtime factors to the total expected productive hours (602 hours), so too should the total maximum potential patient treatments (2,180 treatments, column 18, Table 7.4) be adjusted. Using the 65 percent correction, as was used for hours, and applying this correction to each figure in column 18, results in a total monthly expected number of patient treatments of 1,416. Projected over 12 months, the number of expected patient treatments is 16,992 (rounded to 17,000 in Table 7.3, the Projected Operating Budget).

The expected number of patient treatments provides the first step in establishing fee schedules that take into account the cost of treatment. For example:

1. Average labor cost per treatment

$$\frac{\$18,327 \text{ (column 15, Table 7.4)}}{1,416 \text{ treatments}} = \$12.94/\text{treatment}$$

2. Average total cost per treatment

$$\frac{\$330,239 \text{ (total expenses, Table 7.3)}}{17,000 \text{ treatments}} = \$19.43/\text{treatment}$$

Notice in this example that the average *labor* cost per treatment ($12.94), represents 67 percent of the average *total* cost per treatment ($19.43).

Fee Schedules

The physical therapist administrator has several options in establishing fee schedules. One is to canvas similar departments in the geographical area, find out what the prevailing fees are, and then set or adjust the department's fees accordingly. This approach, of course, ignores any relationship between fees for services and the cost of providing those services. A second option is to adopt a uniform fee (regardless of the kind or amount of treatment) based upon an average total cost per treatment—see, for example, the illustration offered immediately above where this cost was $19.43 per treatment. This second option is certainly better than the first but it could pose a disadvantage for some patients.

The third option is a more precise cost accounting approach. Rodriquez and Rodriquez published such an approach in 1955 (15). Their approach has been used by many. The descriptions and examples that follow represent the author's modification of the Rodriquez and Rodriquez approach (10). There are other approaches for establishing fee schedules, of course, and the reader should consult these sources to compare the different methods of identifying and using cost finding data (6, 8, 9, 13, 14). The author prefers his modified use of Rodriquez and Rodriquez's work, because he feels it minimally fractionalizes the service and yet allows the development of a wide variety of data that can aid in managing a physical therapy service.

The approach to establishing a fee schedule presented here requires the calculation of three different "rates per minute"—a labor cost per productive minute, an overhead cost per minute, and an equipment cost per minute. These three rates are then applied to the appropriate time elements of treatment to determine the total treatment cost. The time elements are taken from a time in motion study by the author. These time elements are illustrative only because they could vary with facilities, personnel, and patients.

Labor Cost per Productive Minute

The reader should refer to the discussion on Productivity, above, where the total expected "productive hours" was calculated to be 602 hours per month for the example physical therapy department; also, in the same place, the labor cost was calculated to be $30.44 per productive hour. The labor cost per productive minute is quite simply:

$$\frac{\$30.44/\text{productive hour}}{60 \text{ minutes}} = \$0.507/\text{productive minute}.$$

In reviewing the previous discussion on Productivity, the reader should recognize that the labor cost identified here includes exployee benefits as well as salaries and wages (column 15, Table 7.4).

Overhead Cost per Minute

From the time the patient enters the department until he leaves, he must bear his share of the department's general overhead. The general overhead includes all direct and indirect expenses *except* salaries and wages and employee benefits (see Table 7.3, Projected Operating Budget). For the physical therapy department as an example, the annual general overhead is:

$ 3,000 Supplies
107,315 Indirect expenses less employee benefits
$110,315 Annual general overhead.

The monthly general overhead is $9,193.

To arrive at the overhead cost per patient per minute, the following chain of calculations is done:

1. Divide the monthly general overhead by 30 days

$$\frac{\$9,193 \text{ overhead/month}}{30 \text{ days}} = \$306.43 \text{ overhead/day}$$

2. Divide the result in step 1 by eight hours

$$\frac{\$306.43 \text{ overhead/day}}{8 \text{ hours}} = \$38.30 \text{ overhead/hour}$$

3. Determine the potential maximum number of patients in the department's space per hour (assume that this number is 15), and take 45 percent of the number (assume that only 45 percent of the potential maximum number of patients will be in the space in a typical hour).

$$15 \text{ patients/hour} \times .45 = 6.75 \text{ patients/hour}$$

4. Divide the result in step 2 by the result in step 3

$$\frac{\$38.30 \text{ overhead/hour}}{6.75 \text{ patients/hour}} = \$5.67 \text{ overhead/patient/hour}$$

5. Divide the result in step 4 by 60 minutes

$$\frac{\$5.67 \text{ overhead/patient/hour}}{60 \text{ minutes}} = \$0.095 \text{ overhead/patient/minute}$$

Equipment Cost per Minute

Calculation of the equipment cost per minute, for professional equipment actually used in patient treatment, requires two considerations: (1) the expected hours of use of any piece of professional equipment in the physical therapy department (this figure will apply uniformly to all professional equipment), and (2) a factor that takes into account the annual depreciation, the maintenance and repair, and the interest on investment for each particular piece of equipment.

The expected hours of use of any piece of equipment is calculated as follows:

1.1. Determine the annual potential hours of use as

$$8 \text{ hours/day} \times 30 \text{ days/month} \times 12 \text{ months} = 2,880 \text{ hours/year}$$

1.2. Determine the annual expected hours of use as a percentage of the potential hours of use (assume that this is 20 percent)

$$2,880 \text{ hours/year} \times .20 = 576 \text{ hours/year expected use.}$$

Now consider some one piece of particular equipment, for example, a whirlpool purchased at $2,000 and with an expected life of five years:

2.1. Determine the annual depreciation

$$\frac{\$2,000 \text{ cost}}{5 \text{ years}} = \$400 \text{ annual depreciation}$$

2.2. Calculate 10 percent of the initial cost for maintenance and repair

$$\$2,000 \text{ cost} \times .10 = \$200 \text{ maintenance and repair}$$

2.3. Calculate 12 percent of the initial cost for interest on investment

$$\$2,000 \text{ cost} \times .12 = \$240 \text{ interest on investment}$$

2.4. Add the results obtained in steps 2.1 through 2.3, and divide the sum by the annual expected hours of use (see step 1.2 above)

$$\frac{\$400 + \$200 + \$240}{576 \text{ hours/year expected use}} = \$1.46 \text{ equipment cost/hour}$$

2.5. Divide the result in step 2.4 by 60 minutes

$$\frac{\$1.46 \text{ equipment cost/hour}}{60 \text{ minutes}} = \$0.024 \text{ equipment cost/minute}$$

Steps 2.1 through 2.5 are applied to any piece of equipment used.

Treatment Cost

To make use of the methods shown above, assume a patient treatment that includes whirlpool, ultrasound, massage, and therapeutic exercises (Orthotron, with table) to the right knee. Assume that the ultrasound initial cost was $1,600 and the Orthotron with table initial cost was $5,000. Assume, also, that each of these devices has an expected life of five years. The equipment cost per minute for the whirlpool, as shown above, is $0.024. The equipment costs per minute for the ultrasound and Orthotron, using steps 2.1 through 2.5 above, are as follows:

Ultrasound ($320 + $160 + $192)/576/60 = $0.019/min.

Orthotron ($1,000 + $500 + $600)/576/60 = $0.061/min.

The reader should work through steps 2.1–2.5 above to verify these calculations.

Given the above equipment costs per minute, the labor cost of $0.507 per productive minute, and the overhead cost per patient per minute of $0.095, see Table 7.6 for a worked example of the total cost of this patient treatment. The total cost of this patient treatment, $27.90, can be compared with the average cost per treatment, $19.43, shown earlier. Both figures were obtained by a cost accounting approach, but the approach used to obtain the result in Table 7.6 is more precise and fairer to patients. The interested reader can use

Table 7.6
Example of Total Treatment Cost

Problem. Calculate the cost of the following physical therapy treatment:
1. Whirlpool to the right knee 20 minutes
2. Ultrasound to the right knee   6 minutes
3. Massage to the right knee 10 minutes
4. Therapeutic exercises to right knee .... 15 minutes

Time Elements in Minutes for This Treatment and Their Proper Assignment

	General Overhead	Equipment	Labor
(1) Whirlpool filled and prepared	0	0	2
(2) Patient stops at reception checks in and checks out	1	0	1
(3) Patient prepares for treatment	2	0	0
(4) Patient put in whirlpool, removed, checked, prepared for ultrasound, massage and exercise	5	0	5
(5) Whirlpool	20	20	0
(6) Ultrasound	6	6	6
(7) Massage	10	0	10
(8) Therapeutic exercises	15	15	15
(9) Whirlpool emptied and cleaned	0	0	2
Totals	59	41	41

	Per Minute Cost	Treatment Time	Treatment Cost
Labor Cost			
Actual time staff is with patient	$0.507 ×	41 min =	$20.79
Equipment Cost			
Actual time equipment is used on patients			
Whirlpool	0.024 ×	20 min =	0.48
Ultrasound	0.019 ×	6 min =	0.11
Orthotron	0.061 ×	15 min =	0.92
Overhead Costs	0.095 ×	59 min =	5.60
Total Treatment Cost			$27.90

the methods and information presented above and in Table 7.6 to see, for example, that a patient treatment consisting of ultrasound only would cost considerably less to provide than the average cost per treatment of $19.43.

Profit Margin

The cost of the treatment is probably not what the fee for the service would be. How much should be added to the treatment cost for profit? What is profit? Should there be a profit? What is reasonable? Who defines what is reasonable? Profit, in fiscal matters, is the monetary gain or benefit in excess of costs from making or providing something. Nonprofit organizations can only seek to recover their costs. However, most businesses and professionals expect to make a profit from their efforts and investments. When manufacturing products, it is customary to set the selling price at five times the cost of the product. Frequently the selling price is discounted 40 percent to stores or dealers. The remaining 60 percent is lessened by the other costs of doing business, i.e., providing capital, carrying inventory, promoting, marketing, etc. Contractors in the building trades routinely pass on to the buyer double their labor costs. They too have to support costs for their business that erode their margin of profit.

Professionals charge for their services in a wide variety of ways. Most of them do not have formulas that specifically fix costs for their professional services. Many times their fees are set during periods of low or medium productivity and it is only after becoming successful and busy that their incomes increase. Many professionals feel this is as it should be because of the long hours of work they have to put in plus the advance educational requirements and the long time necessary to attain success. Whatever the profits they reap from their activities, almost all feel they are entitled to what they receive. In fact, the quest for economic reward has made this country the success it is today. Health professional services are the result of advanced education, assumption of responsibility, and the professional's accountability for his or her actions. The health professional also must be skillful in handling personal crises, be on demand call, and give a large investment of time and money. Certainly, the percentage of return for such effort should be more than the interest rates on money. A reasonable profit should take into consideration all factors and be relative to whatever standards are practiced in the other segments of society.

OTHER FACTORS AFFECTING FISCAL MANAGEMENT

Economic Philosophy of the Facility

Cost accounting methods allow a candid examination of the factors necessary to produce the physical therapy service. However, there are other factors that will affect the fiscal management of a physical therapy practice. Since all costs of the service have to be paid, the economic philosophy of the provider must establish whether or not the service will be philanthropic, nonprofit, for profit, or a combination of philanthropic and nonprofit and for profit. This philosophy will have great impact on the emphasis that must be placed upon controlling expenses and securing income.

Community Needs

The size, age, and employment characteristics of the community have important bearing on potential physical therapy patient caseloads. If the community is small, made up mostly of young people whose employment does not require much physical work output, the potential physical therapy caseload would be expected to be small. If the community is large, with more adults and older people who work at various jobs that require a variety of physical activity, the potential physical therapy caseload would be expected to be larger. Historically, the geographic area, its economy, and the variety of patient pathology in the community have great effect upon the demand for physical therapy services.

Kinds of Services Offered

The kinds of services to be offered will influence all aspects of management. The personnel needs, physical plant, equipment, and administrative structure of the service will vary widely depending upon several variables. These variables include: 1) the nature of the clinical services provided (e.g., general, rehabilitative, or specialized); 2) the educational functions of the service (clinical education for students, in-service education for other professionals and health workers, and education of the community); 3) the consultative responsibilities of the staff; and 4) the research activities of the service.

Utilization Patterns of Referring Physicians

The utilization patterns of referring physicians will have great effect upon clinical facilities. These patterns will reflect the physicians' specialties, treatment philosophy, and knowledge of physical therapy.

Patient Volume, Days and Hours of Service

The kinds and volume of patient pathology will have much to do with the size and mix of personnel as well as the size of the department and equipment needed. The hours and days of service will also be important to know and to plan for.

Sophistication of the Facility

The sophistication of the facility or provider will also have great bearing on fiscal management. Such things as the cost of computers, size of hallways and reception areas, class of building construction, methods of cost allocation, numbers of administrative staff, details of data retreival, etc., will all add costs that are indirectly considered part of the costs to be shared by the physical therapy department.

Contracted Versus Employed Physical Therapy Staff

It is estimated that 75 percent of all physical therapy departments in the United States of America employ their physical therapy personnel and that the other 25 percent contract with physical therapists to supply the physical therapy service. Most physical therapy contractors supply personnel, but frequently the contractors also supply other elements of the physical therapy service such as equipment and supplies. Most contractors believe that they have a stronger voice professionally and economically in providing the service and therefore have more motivation to control the availability, quality and quantity of the physical therapy service. This can be true. However, if both the employed physical therapist and the contractor are equally skilled, both professionally and businesswise, and are equally motivated, there should be no difference in the quality, quantity and the availability of the service.

Because of the very nature of a contract, the contractor operates under incentives to hold down the costs of providing services and at the same time to increase both the quality and quantity of those services. The contract also allows the physical therapy administrator the potential opportunity to personally earn an amount of income that is more commensurate with others of similar skills and knowledge; additionally, his earnings can be more directly related to success as both a professional and a business person. Usually, contractors earn more money than salaried physical therapists (3, 4). Some health facilities are almost forced to use contractors because they do not have enough patient load to warrant a full time physical therapist, or because they may be in a geographic area where physical therapists are not available as employees, or because the available physical therapists do not have the knowledge, skill or interest to develop or manage a physical therapy service.

Salary Equivalency

Salary equivalency is a term used to identify regulations promulgated by the Department of Health and Human Services (HHS, formerly, the Department of Health, Education, and Welfare) to control or regulate the amount of money that the Medicare program will pay health facilities for physical therapy services supplied by a physical therapy contractor. The regulations establish an hourly rate for each state called the *adjusted hourly salary equivalency amount* (AHSEA). The AHSEA is established by using figures collected every three years by the U.S. Department of Labor's Bureau of Labor Statistics (BLS) plus a 50 percent addition of the salary amount for fringe benefits and other expenses. The BLS survey compiles the hourly wages paid to staff (nonsupervisory) physical therapists who are employed by certain hospitals. The HHS uses the BLS figures to develop each state's AHSEA and then periodically updates the AHSEA by an inflation factor.

The AHSEA is applied to all hours that the contractor provides on-site services to a facility. Medicare reimburses the facility only for the hours spent on Medicare patients in ratio to all patients. The system requires more record keeping and auditing than when the physical therapy service is supplied by employees of the health care facility. A log must be maintained to identify the on-site regular and overtime hours of the physical therapy staff including the department head, supervisors, staff physical therapists, physical therapist assistants, and physical therapy aides. The department heads and supervisors are not reimbursed for overtime hours. Additionally, days worked at the site must be recorded in a log. A record must also be available to identify equipment depreciation and cost of supplies if they are supplied by the contractor. Adjustments are made in the AHSEA when it is applied to physical therapist assistants, supervisors, and to overtime hours. The government's definition of a supervisor and how many people must be supervised affects the hourly rate allowed for supervision. Records must also be kept to identify who treats each patient and how many of the patients are Medicare patients. The records are audited annually three to six months after the close of the fiscal year. After the audit, the government will pay either the actual cost or the costs figured on the AHSEA formula, whichever is less. If the health facility has paid the physical therapy contractor more than the identified allowed costs, Medicare will not reimburse the health facility any amount over the Medicare percentage of the total costs. "If the health facility has been paid more than the allowed costs for Medicare patients, it must rebate the difference to the government."

The salary equivalency system contains several other inequities. Among these are:

1. If an employed physical therapist's staff personnel costs are higher than a contractor's, the employed physical therapist's staffed facility can be reimbursed for actual cost. The contractor's personnel costs are strictly limited by the AHSEA.

2. The system does not account for all hours that a contractor may legitimately spend administering a department. Physical therapy personnel employed by a health facility can, but the contractor cannot, be paid for any off-site time or effort spent working on behalf of the physical therapy department or health care facility.

3. The AHSEA does not realistically take into account all costs. The system allows an expense factor of 50 percent of salary to be reimbursed for fringe benefits and other expenses. The expenses in running a physical therapy department cannot be recouped by adding 50 percent to the salary costs.

4. The definition of supervisor does not reflect the actual practice of physical therapy. The HHS requires an individual to supervise five physical therapists before that individual can be reimbursed the full supervisory amount. The HHS will not reimburse for supervising aides, physical therapist assistants or other nonphysical therapists. The amounts reimbursed for supervision are clearly too low as evidenced by the BLS survey for 1978 (5).

5. The record-keeping system is complex, duplicative, time-consuming, and costly.

6. The AHSEA amounts are consistently and grossly out of date. As of July 1, 1980, for example, the AHSEA's were based on a BLS survey taken in 1975 and updated in October, 1978, based on an inflation factor calculated as of April, 1978. The AHSEA as of July 1, 1980 was at least 26 months out of date.

The American Physical Therapy Association (APTA) has opposed the use of the salary equivalency system since its inception. The APTA has offered on many occasions (to no avail) alternative methods of cost containment that encourage productivity, reduction of costs, and correction of the inequalities to the patient, the physical therapy profession, the health care facilities, and the taxpayers. The APTA has attempted to persuade HHS to change the procedures used to determine reimbursement under salary equivalency in order to solve some of the inequities discussed above. A system must be arrived at that encourages productivity and in so doing returns a fair compensation to the physical therapist. Paying for hours worked at a rate less than the hourly cost of working does neither.

Productivity—Another Look

Productivity is defined as a physical therapist's ability to produce income by patient care, including evaluation, treatment planning, and patient education.

Productivity is so important to fiscal management that a more detailed presentation of some of the factors that affect productivity is warranted.

Down Time

Down time is the time that an employee's availability to be productive is infringed upon. Some of the factors are constant and some are intermittent. Some facilities report as little as 20 percent and others report more than 50 percent. The constant factors depend upon the facility's particular requirements; the intermittent factors can fluctuate widely. Down time factors can limit the employee's productivity by 35 percent so that they can only be 65 percent maximally productive. Some of these factors are:

1. Statutory and customary breaks, i.e., coffee, etc.
2. Abbreviated work days (less than eight hours a day is available because of getting ready to start and getting ready to stop work at the beginning of the day, before and after breaks, before and after lunch, and at the end of the day)
3. Consultations with department heads, other physical therapists, physicians, nurses, other medical workers, patients, and patient families
4. Record keeping for evaluations, treatment plans, daily notes, weekly summaries, discharge summaries, progress reports and letters to physicians and third party payers, and other Medicare Fiscal Intermediaries' requirements
5. In-service education for physical therapy staff and other staff of the facility
6. Teaching commitments—teaching student physical therapists, attending educational meetings, writing student programs, writing student evaluations
7. Indirect administrative activities
   a. Departmental organization meetings
   b. Collecting department statistics
   c. Planning and developing new programs
   d. Constructive discussions relative to current departmental services
   e. Personnel activities
   f. Participating in meetings within and outside the facility, e.g., utili-

zation review, safety, facility department heads, and employee benefit committees community relations programs, etc.

8. Patient nonavailability
   a. No show: patient does not cancel or keep appointment
   b. Cancellation of treatment: patient cancels appointment
   c. Patient not available: patient being treated by physician or other
      department within the facility
9. Transportation lags: applicable to the physical therapist going to the
   patient or the patient coming to the therapist
   a. Slow elevators
   b. Time necessary to find transportation equipment
   c. Travel time to the patient or department
   d. Patient late for treatment because of transportation complications
      or patient not being ready for transport

Obviously, this list of down time factors could include other factors and
the impact of any one or combination of down time factors can be expected
to vary from facility to facility and from time to time.

Department Management

Usually the director is the highest paid professional in the department.
Salary is commensurate with experience, skill, effectiveness, and size of the
facility and its staff. The director, or his equivalent, is not usually involved
in direct patient care and is mostly responsible for staff, staff supervision,
and:

1. Purpose of department;
2. Organizational plan;
3. Administrative procedures;
4. Documentation and data retrieval;
5. Co-ordination of patient care;
6. Fiscal management;
7. Adequacy of physical therapy plant and equipment;
8. Co-ordination of continuing education of staff.

Supervision

The supervisory needs of a physical therapy service are dependent upon
one or a combination of all of the following: the kinds of patient pathology,
the volume and mix of the patient load, the number and training of the
personnel working in the service, the personnel's productive capacity, and
the quality of the service. Some professionals feel that five people should be
the maximum number of people that any one supervisor can effectively
supervise and still be expected to produce quality work. Universally acceptable supervision standards for physical therapy departments do not yet exist.
Obviously, the fewer people supervised by one supervisor, the higher the

supervisory cost; and the more people supervised by one supervisor, the lower the supervisory cost. An APTA Salary Survey in 1973 showed that physical therapy department head salaries averaged 50 percent greater than staff physical therapist salaries (3). The salaries of supervisors below department heads averaged 35 percent greater than staff physical therapists' salaries. Other studies report supervisor salary ratios to be 20 to 60 percent greater than staff physical therapy salaries (16). The 1978 Bureau of Labor Statistics salary survey for hospitals reports supervisory salary differentials to be from 18 to 62 percent greater than staff physical therapy salaries (5). The author believes that if a physical therapist assumes the responsibilities of managing a one-man physical therapy department, that therapist should be paid an amount in addition to what that therapist should receive for treating patients.

Physician's Services

If a physician's services are used in a physical therapy department and compensated through the department's operating budget, the department's labor cost per productive hour will be affected but not the number of patient treatments. The physician does not render direct physical therapy patient care.

Clerical, Reception, General Office and Secretarial Personnel

These categories of personnel are absolutely necessary to assist in the professional and business activities of the physical therapy department. The number of them needed will be influenced by the size and variety of the patient load, the staff and the services of the department, and the size and location of the department.

"The support efforts of these personnel, like the leadership and directive efforts of personnel responsible for department management and supervision, affect the productivity of physical therapists. These efforts must be considered as expenses of the service, and obviously income must be generated to pay for such expenses."

CONCLUSIONS

Fiscal management is a science and an art. If the physical therapist administrator is to be successful in fiscal management, he must have, or understand, the necessary skills and be able to blend the science and art of economics with professional knowledge and skills to the end that the physical therapy department and its service are not compromised. Expenses and income should be managed so that the physical therapy services are of high quality, in enough quantity, and available to all at a reasonable cost.

References

1. American Hospital Association: Budgeting procedures of hospitals. Chicago, 1961.
2. American Hospital Association: Chart of accounts for hospitals. Chicago, 1966.

3. American Physical Therapy Association: Income survey of membership. Insert in Progress Report, membership news APTA, *3:* (8), 1974.
4. American Physical Therapy Association: Membership profile survey—A summary report. Insert in Progress Report, membership news APTA, *8:* (1), 1979.
5. Bureau of Labor Statistics: Excerpts from industry wage survey—Hospitals, Various major metropolitan areas. U.S. Department of Labor, Bureau of Labor Statistics, Washington, 1978.
6. Burton, B., Hewitt, D.R., Patten, F.L., Graves, D.A., Magistro, C.M., and McKillip, J.B.: Guidelines for the establishment of fees for physical therapy services. J. Am. Phys. Ther. Assoc., *45:* 730–7y33, 1965.
7. California Hospital Association: Uniform cost accounting manual. Sacramento, 1964.
8. Gee, D.A., and Hickok, R.J.: Cost analysis development for a department. J. Am. Phys. Ther. Assoc., *42:* 383–387, 1962.
9. Gee, D.A., and Hickok, R.J.: Developing unit costs for physical therapy modalities. J. Am. Phys. Ther. Assoc., *42:* 713–718, 1962.
10. McKillip, J.B.: Criteria for developing physical therapy fee schedules. J. Am. Phys. Ther. Assoc., *42:* 303–306, 1962.
11. McKillip, J.B.: Planning the physical therapy department—Fiscal aspects. J. Am. Phys. Ther. Assoc., *45:* 1175–1178, 1965.
12. McKillip, J.B., and Dicus, R.G.: Cost analysis and cost accounting. Phys. Ther., *51:* 79–80, 1971.
13. Price, J.W.: Setting rates for physical therapy services. Phys. Ther., J. Am. Phys. Ther. Assoc., *49:* 265–268, 1969.
14. Ramsden, E.L., and Fisher, W.T.: Cost allocation for physical therapy in a teaching hospital. Phys. Ther., J. Am. Phys. Ther. Assoc., *50:* 660–664, 1970.
15. Rodriquez, A.A., and Rodriquez, A.: Schedule of charges for physical therapy services. Phy. Ther. Rev., *35:* 295–298, 1955.
16. Valley Presbyterian Hospital Survey of Supervisor Salary Differential in Like Facilities in Southern California (unpublished), 1980. Available from James B. McKillip, RPT, 15243 Vanowen St., 102, Van Nuys, CA 91405.

INDEX